MANMADE™

MANMADE™

THE ESSENTIAL SKINCARE & GROOMING REFERENCE FOR EVERY MAN

CHRIS SALGARDO

PRESIDENT, KIEHL'S SINCE 1851

PAM KRAUSS BOOKS
NEW YORK

Pam Krauss Books and colophon are trademarks of Penguin Random House LLC.
Manmade is a trademark of Manmade, LLC.
The apothecary K (symbol) is a trademark of L'OREAL USA Creative, Inc.

Library of Congress Cataloging-in-Publication Data is available upon request.

ISBN 978-0-8041-8697-1
eBook ISBN 978-0-8041-8698-8

Printed in the United States of America

Book design by Eleanor Safe and Bruce Burton, Davis® Brand Capital
Cover design by Eleanor Safe and Bruce Burton, Davis® Brand Capital

Photo credits: p. 10 (Anthony Mackie) Tommaso Boddi/Getty Images; pp. 14, 19, 22, 95,
121, 147, 179, 207, and 234 (Chris Salgardo) Travis Shinn; p. 88 (Teddy Sears) Rainer
Hosch; p. 116 (Paul Cox) JJ Sulin; p. 140 (Grant Reynolds) Travis Shinn; p. 160 (Tattoo
Gun/Hand) Shawn Connell; p. 165 (Tattoo Body) Craig Paulson; p. 166 (Chef Paul)
Evan Sung; p. 172 (Jaytech) Kristján Czakó; p. 200 (Jake Barton) Atlantic Monthly

10 9 8 7 6 5 4 3 2 1

First Edition

For my parents, Ken and Lorene,
for guiding me toward the man I am today

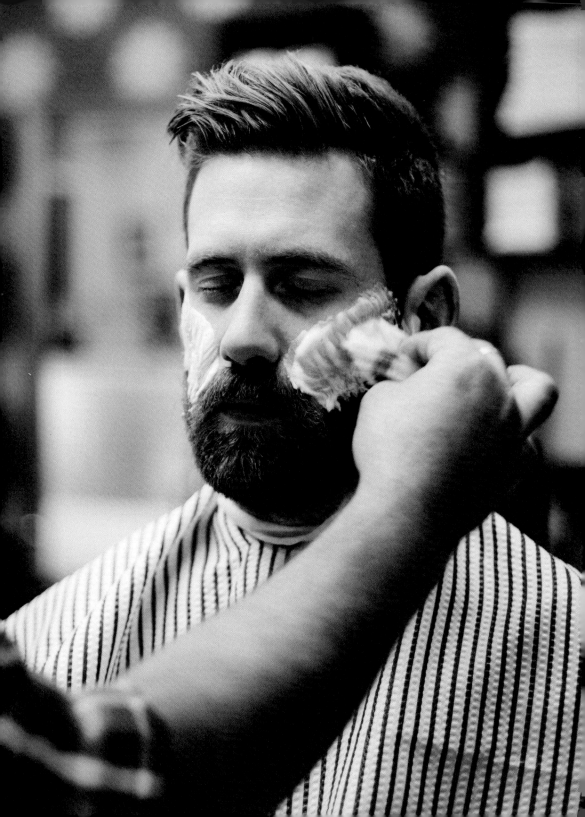

CONTENTS

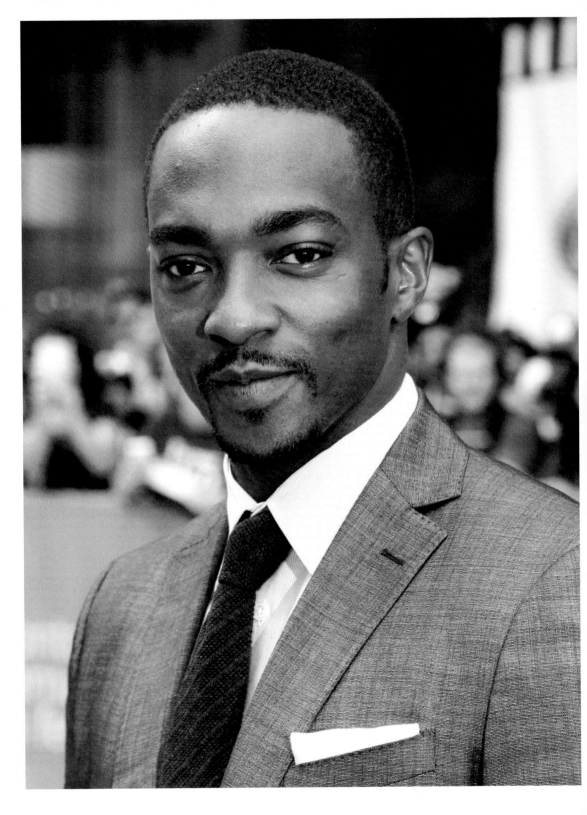

FOREWORD
BY ANTHONY MACKIE

From cleanliness and purity, good things can grow.

I have found this to be true in all aspects of life: my love, my family, my career, my philanthropy. For me, getting rid of all the noise, the distraction, and the dirt of life makes everything else possible. As a man, doing so is a commitment to those I love. As an actor, it is essential to what I do when I transform myself for a role. As a citizen of this planet, it is how I keep my promise of shared respect and stewardship of where we all live.

So in my life, being a *man* is about finding ways to achieve a clean mind, spirit, and body. Caring for myself is how I prepare to care for and connect with others. It isn't just a ritual I go through, it is a philosophy I live by. It may be tempting to see skincare and grooming as nothing more than necessary tasks, but they *are* more than that. They are, very often, our first intentional acts of the day—the moments when we focus and decide how to present ourselves to the world.

At least that is how I see it: "getting ready" is really about "becoming ready"—focused, prepared—for what is to come. Life can be tough, random, even chaotic at times. We all have to put on our game faces—our best—and push through it. That's why I think a book like this matters.

Of course, like so many men, I had to learn how to care for myself and what it meant to do so properly. It wasn't part of how I grew up. My dad worked construction for forty years, and used no more than a bar of soap at the end of workdays. End of story. No SPF for his hours out in the sun. No moisturizer to help his skin recover while he slept. No hand salve to ease the wear of labor. Believe it or not, I grew up not even aware that as an African American I could get a sunburn (and, wow, was the first one was a doozy).

There was a lot to learn along the way to where life has taken me. I did not even know what to buy, nor where to buy it. I followed the advice of experts, Chris Salgardo among them. And I soon ended up realizing that by caring for myself with intention I looked better, felt better, and presented myself to others with more focus.

You don't have to be in the public eye to take your grooming and skin-care seriously. And doing it right doesn't have to be a big deal. For me, it is part of the job—but it is also part of my life. It does not matter what type of guy you are—maybe polished and professional, maybe rugged and carefree. We all benefit from taking just a few minutes to ready ourselves for the world before us.

For younger men, getting the basics right early on will help more than I can tell you. You will be protecting your skin, finding what works best, and feeling confident sooner in life. My six-year-old son loves the time we spend getting the dirt to go away and making all things bright and fresh. He is incredibly keen on being "put together" and looking good at school. From this clean place, I know he can grow into anybody he dreams of being.

No, there is no secret potion—but yes, there is a bit of magic that comes when we decide to care about the details. It is how we show respect for ourselves and those around us. This book will help you do that, no matter who you are now or may become throughout your life.

When I first met Chris Salgardo at an event in Los Angeles, I confided in him that I finally understood why skincare and grooming mattered—far beyond just that bar of soap my dad used. We became great friends. I hope you will benefit from his insights and wisdom here as much as I have.

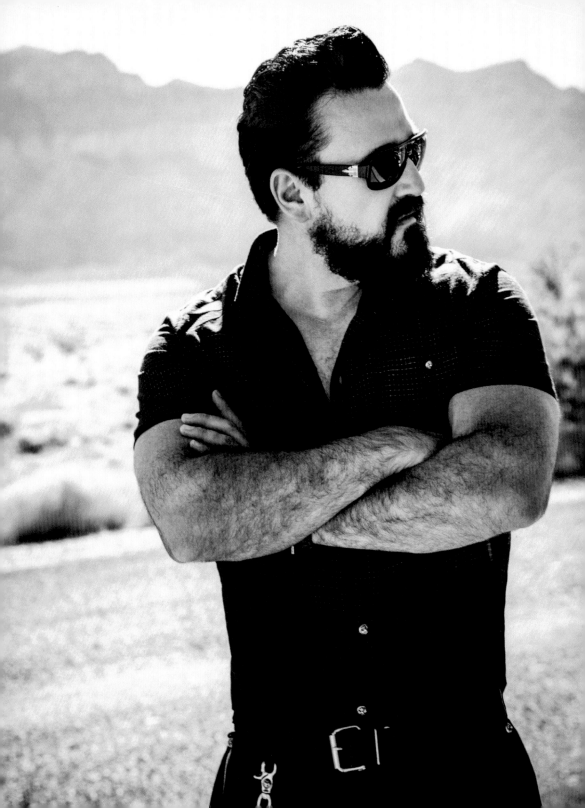

INTRODUCTION

A friend of mine recently sat his wife down and announced that there was something he needed to say regarding their two-year-old son. It was important, he emphasized. Looking her straight in the eye, he said, without a drop of irony, *"If anything should ever happen to me . . . tell Jake to moisturize."*

While he was only partly in earnest, my friend was doing something that few fathers do—or have done. He was sharing the knowledge about personal care and grooming he had learned through trial and error. Yes, moisturizing really matters. It protects the skin, keeping your largest organ (sorry, guys, it's true) hydrated, healthy, and in balance. Without it, ironically, you can end up with not only dry skin but a buildup of oil that any Texas wildcatter would happily lay claim to. I'm here to help you avoid that. Jake has the benefit of good advice from his father, but like most men I've met since taking the helm at Kiehl's Since 1851 in the U.S., I bet you still have questions. Lots of them.

There was a long journey of learning what worked for me: how to feel confident, even as a pimply kid; what my skin really needed to be healthy and not be damaged by the sun when I became a bike enthusiast; why caring for my body would serve me well throughout my life.

The simple truth is: The basics of skincare and grooming don't get passed along by the other men in our lives—whether fathers, big brothers, coaches, or even skincare experts. It was somehow all just supposed to be known—by osmosis, from watching TV, flipping through magazines, or by trial and error. Before I came to lead one of the most successful and iconic brands in skincare, the sum total of my skincare and grooming education was a single pronouncement from my father: Use an electric razor. Nothing about preparing my face before shaving or protecting it after. Not unlike mowing the lawn, the goal was straightforward: fire it up and run over anything that seems too long. And as far as the other hair on my face—like eyebrows, or nose or ear hair—forget about it. Not a word. His advice got me out of the gates, but that was about it.

There was a long journey of learning what worked for me: how to feel confident, even as a pimply kid; what my skin really needed to be healthy and not be damaged by the sun when I became a bike enthusiast; why caring for my body would serve me well throughout my life. It wasn't Dad's fault—personal care for men simply wasn't the practice at that time. But times and practices have changed.

Today there is a new level of expectation: No matter what type of man you might be, it's smart, not narcissistic, to take care of yourself, to take pride in your appearance, and to be mindful about your grooming. Whether your personal style is formal or relaxed, good, practical knowledge can help you get to your best self on every front. At the end of the day it's not really about appearance (at least not exclusively about that); it's a matter of protecting your skin and solving problems when they come up. I hope this book will address the unanswered questions you may have about grooming and make a good case for treating your skin, hair, and appearance with the respect they deserve. It's a manual I would have loved to have had earlier in my life and career. Based on the questions I field every day, I'm guessing I'm not the only one.

Nearly everywhere I go, in fact, I'm approached by men seeking out advice: at the gym while working out, at a social event to support one of my charitable efforts, walking down the street after a TV appearance, or while opening a new Kiehl's store and shaking hands. It doesn't matter where or when—the questions keep coming my way, often from men so polished and put together, you would think they already had all the answers. Or from the "man's man" who, outwardly, seems not to care about wrinkles (facial or sartorial). Or from younger men—skateboarders or cyclists—who know that sunscreen matters but are confused by body image pressures and manscaping expectations. Or from the creative-genius night owls whose workplaces are clubs or kitchens or studios—and whose complexions are pallid as a result. I've been asked by titans of industry—men who could outthink and out-deal us all—how to feel "less geeky" and look better in middle age. We all want to feel confident and healthy and attractive in our own ways. These are the concerns that have shaped this book.

As I was preparing to write this book for today's men, I gathered groups of them to ask the questions I had been pondering: What were you taught and by whom? How did you learn what you needed to know? What do you think is most important for men to know? Turns out, those questions were just the tip of the iceberg. The more I listened, the more questions surfaced.

The discussion—both the questions and the answers—was surprising. Though we all had very little in common as individuals, our collective

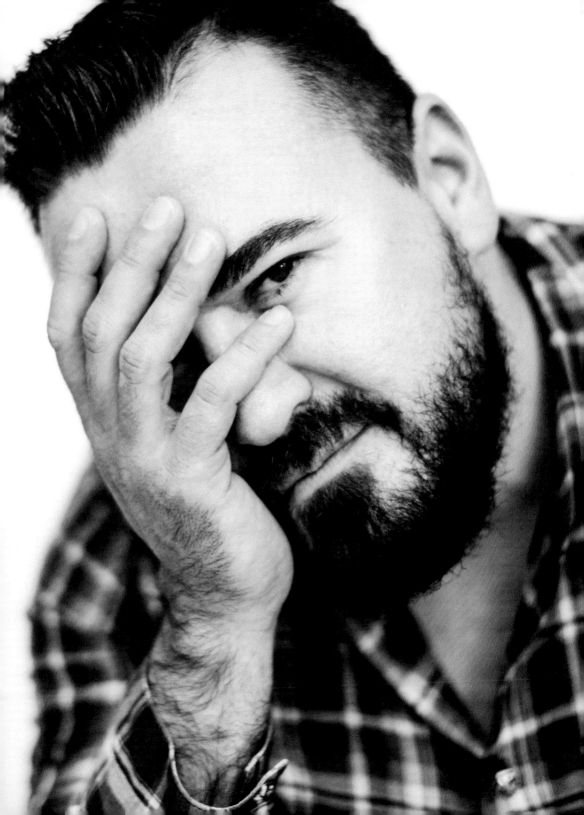

experience was strikingly similar. Across men aged twenty-five to fifty-five, whether polished professionals or down-to-earth guys—married, single, gay, straight—not one of us had been taught to shave by our dads. That's not to say we haven't developed our own grooming rituals, skincare practices, and strong preferences. With few exceptions the guys I spoke with disliked products with added or heavy fragrances, and used lip balm regularly. So you read it here first: Today's man taught himself how to shave, smells naturally clean, and has soft lips. Not a bad start, all things considered, but hardly the end of the story.

The men I spoke with were hardly indifferent to grooming matters, they were just at a loss as to where to turn for guidance. Some reported learning what worked best from their friends, others picked up things here and there—maybe a tip from a barber or something they heard or read. But mostly, their knowledge of skincare and grooming had been casual and cultural—observed, but not taught, per se. The answers haven't all been in one place, and men have had to search things out and do the best they could, adapting these little nuggets to fit their circumstances, life stage, and lifestyle as best they could—sometimes with decidedly mixed results.

I wrote this book to help move the discussion forward, and to do so in the way that men like to learn—by reporting on what others are doing. Mostly, though, I want to share the wisdom I have garnered from decades at the top of the skincare industry—from working directly with men on their everyday challenges, creating breakthrough products with scientists, and developing effective treatments with dermatologists. I want to share this knowledge with you, and apply it through the real-life needs of different types of men. I want to share the questions, concerns, stories, and habits of some remarkable men, and translate their solutions into tools you can add to your own arsenal. And I want to give some simple advice, life hacks, and survival tips too, so you're never without the ability to look and feel your very best—no matter what type of life you are designing for yourself. This is not a one-size-fits-all approach—nor is it a platform to push products. This is about real problems, practical solutions, reliable knowledge, and what works best for you.

While I reject the notion of the "ideal" modern man, a single archetype we should all aspire to, after speaking to literally thousands of customers, friends, and folks in the fashion and beauty world, I've identified a few broad categories representative of the real men I meet and interact with every day: the Modern Polished Gentleman, the Hands-On Guy, the Extreme Dude, the Artistic Rebel, and the Renaissance Man. Perhaps you can relate to one of these categories—or several. We are each different types of men at different times. Who you are and how you present yourself on vacation or in your downtime might bear little resemblance to the image you project during work hours. All of us—at one time or another—need to know how to be our gentlemanly best. We need to care for ourselves in one way when pushing the limits through winter sports, and in another way as we shift perspectives on what matters and what we will create in this life. We need to counteract the toll

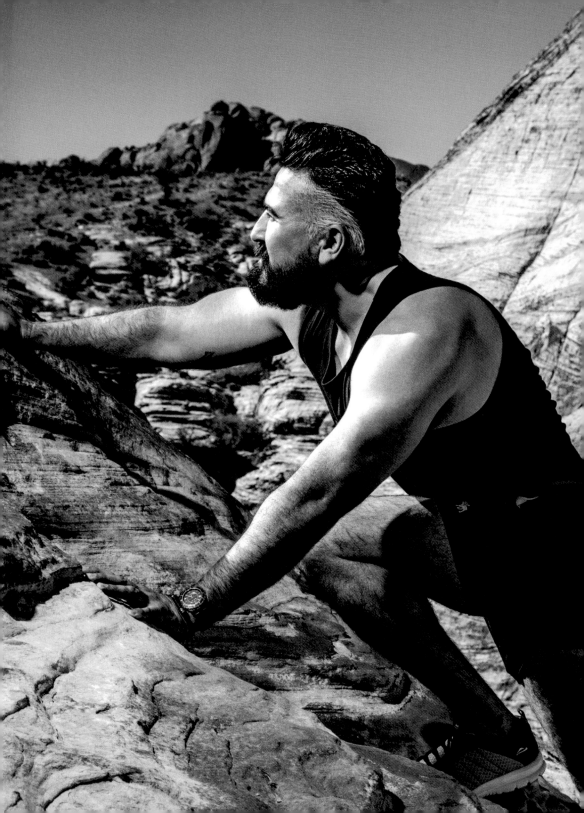

that travel and work may take on us, whether that means spending time in a car and an office, or airports and hotels. While there is no one way of being a man today, there is definitely a right way to practice skincare and grooming.

So let's start with some context to set the stage, a few basics in terms of techniques, and then some real-world questions that may sound like your own. My goal here is to demystify skincare and grooming, and to help you refocus on real-world questions and answers that will give you the tools to put your best face forward every single day, no matter where that day takes you. You may not need all the advice offered here, but at least some of it will resonate. I promise you that.

Whoever you are—or are becoming—as a man, I am here to help you care for yourself, and look and feel the very best you can. It's your life. It should be **MANMADE**.

Chris LaGanla

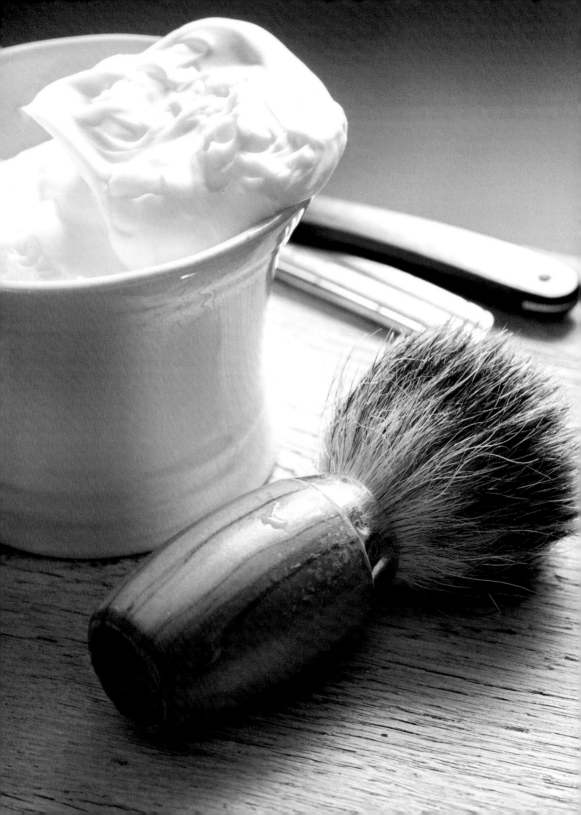

PART I

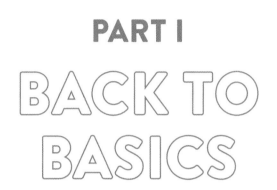

BACK TO
BASICS

GROOMING
PRIMER

1

YOUR LITTLE BLACK BOOK FOR LOOKING YOUR BEST

A golden age of grooming is upon us. Over the past few years a wealth of products, treatments, and procedures—some of which I've been responsible for—have hit the market, and the truth is, it can all be a bit overwhelming. There's advice coming from every direction and new "secret tips" from self-proclaimed experts every day. Skincare and grooming specialty shops for men seem to be popping up on every corner. This can leave us wondering what is necessary, what is a waste, and who to trust. *Does using a badger hair shaving brush, in fact, make a difference? And eye cream—what exactly does it do, and how?*

How many times have you walked into an interesting store or looked at an intriguing product only to leave empty-handed and feeling baffled or sheepish? Our fathers and their fathers before them managed to get by with nothing but the most basic grooming products, so do we really need to rethink our serum strategy? The answer is "yes," with a side of "no." The options, while plentiful, must be manageable, practical, effective, and, above all, efficient. This isn't about making things more complex. It's about learning what will work best for you, your life, and your skin—and on *your* schedule.

The man who revels in the ceremony of an old-school, straight-razor hot shave isn't necessarily the same man who is racing against the clock each morning with exactly ten minutes to get out the door. What might be a required weekly ritual for one guy might be a twice-yearly indulgence for another. Taking care of yourself doesn't have to be very involved. "Keeping it simple" doesn't have to translate into "letting things go." It's all a matter of being intentional and precise with the selection of products arranged on your sink top, inside your medicine chest, or tucked into your Dopp kit. What's right for you on a busy workday compared to a fun weekend away with friends or family? What's the difference between a regular Monday morning recovery regimen and the one required after too much fun in the sun? This isn't about being fussy. It's about looking your best and feeling great.

Taking care of yourself often sounds easier said than done, and there's a reason why that is true. It's taken thousands and thousands of years to learn what works, invent what's needed, and create a regimen that is both realistic and effective. So, how did we get to today's habits, and what do you really need to know about them? Let's take a brief historical tour of men's grooming and skincare.

Long before the days of $150 haircuts—or walk-in, strip-mall cuts, for that matter—there were the primates. There is no shortage of YouTube videos and nature documentaries dedicated to the intricate cleaning and grooming habits of these fine creatures. And much like the humans that followed, when primates engage in the act of *allogrooming,* or "social grooming," there is much more happening than meets the eye. Each mat untangled and clump of dirt removed represents a social construct—a firmly established and critical bond. The relationships aren't romantic; it's purely friend stuff.

Learning to take care of ourselves was taught, passed forward, woven into our DNA. Luckily, these days we have barbers, stylists, skincare experts, and loved ones to help us with the rituals that will make us look and feel good.

More than a few evolutionary and historical steps later came the Egyptians—and they changed everything. Unlike the civilizations before them, the Egyptians associated hair and skin maintenance with class and wealth. Cleopatra and Queen Nefertiti planted the seeds of present-day manicures, employing extravagant oils and henna dyes on their hands and feet. Kohl was used by both men and women to define and highlight the eyes. Egyptians concocted oils and creams to shield their faces and bodies from the hot African sun as far back as 3000 BC. Men made blades of flint or pumice stone and used them to keep their faces smooth and clean. The Egyptians even developed a process for removing hair using sugar. Thus, a nation of manscapers was born, long before it debuted on modern reality television.

Fast-forward a few thousand years and we arrive at the time of Alexander the Great, who famously required his soldiers to be clean-

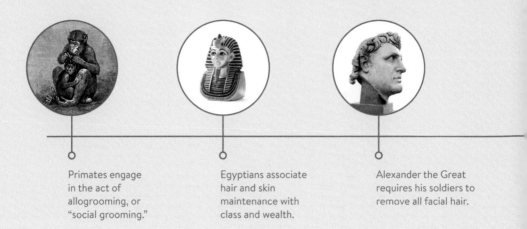

Primates engage in the act of allogrooming, or "social grooming."

Egyptians associate hair and skin maintenance with class and wealth.

Alexander the Great requires his soldiers to remove all facial hair.

shaven, so that their enemies could not grab their beards in combat. Would the Western World as we know it exist if not for this strategic decision? We'll never know. What we do know is that grooming was starting to be seen for its practical, even life-saving benefits, not just as a means of social bonding or indication of status.

Around AD 100, the men of Rome took their skincare game to the next level—by developing oils and creams to cover blemishes and smooth skin, and going as far as to polish their nails with sheep's blood and fat. The Romans, who were well regarded for their lavish bathhouses and rituals, created their own mud baths. They filled large tubs with a unique and frankly unappealing blend of dirt and crocodile excrement. How far we've come in what to expect from a "spa experience."

In the relatively more recent sixteenth and seventeenth centuries, powdered wigs, or perukes, were all the rage in Europe, and with good reason. Syphilis was rampant at that time, and in more advanced stages

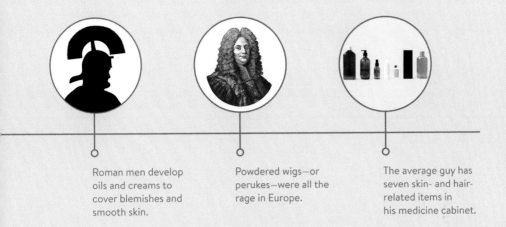

Roman men develop oils and creams to cover blemishes and smooth skin.

Powdered wigs—or perukes—were all the rage in Europe.

The average guy has seven skin- and hair-related items in his medicine cabinet.

the disease causes patchy hairlessness. A lush wig complete with flowing ringlets and voluminous curls spared the afflicted from public scrutiny and embarrassment. Those who suffered male-pattern baldness also quickly jumped on the wig bandwagon, thanks to the influence of the teenaged Louis XIV and his rapidly balding head. English barbers were soon promoted to esteemed positions in the royal courts. The style fell out of fashion by the late eighteenth century, however, supplanted by a more natural, less costume-like look. Skincare and grooming had taken on the broadest cultural import, signaling health, wealth, and power.

And so we arrive at the present, still with plenty of questions to ask and lessons to learn about how best to present ourselves to the world. While many of our grooming practices are steeped in tradition, with thousands of years of history on their side, grooming for men has faded from elaborate ritual or a survivalist's necessity to a near afterthought. At the end of the day, there should be community, comfort, and connection when it comes to how we take care of ourselves as men. Instead,

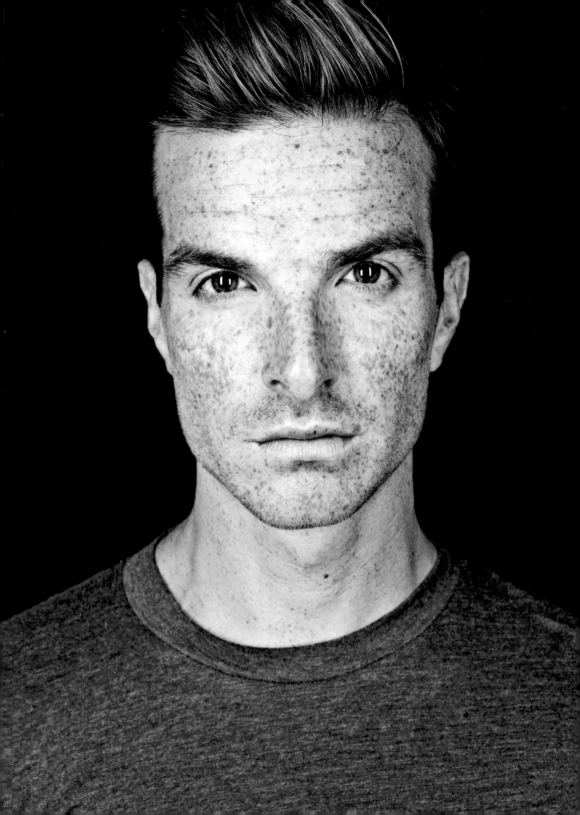

We are none of us unevolved apes, idealized soldiers of empires past, nor dandyish courtiers. We are, simply, men.

there is a sense, too often, of needing "permission" to ask questions and learn the basics. If you have questions, you've come to the right place. But first, a few for you.

Is a rockabilly, retro-chic aesthetic your go-to look? Or do you seek a high-performance, tech-savvy patina? Is a smooth, clean face your go-to look, or have you been contemplating something edgier? These days there are so many opportunities for self-expression, and within all these looks there is a well-groomed aesthetic that tells the world you care about how you are perceived and received.

Today, a smart skincare and grooming regimen is an integral part of every guy's overall presentation. Why invest in a sharp wardrobe if the head and shoulders supporting it don't look equally well-tended? Some men have clearly already gotten that message—the average guy has seven skin- and hair-related items in his medicine cabinet. Whether or not he knows precisely what to do with those products is another matter entirely. And if you're not quite there yet, it's my job to show you the way. I promise you will like what you see on the other side.

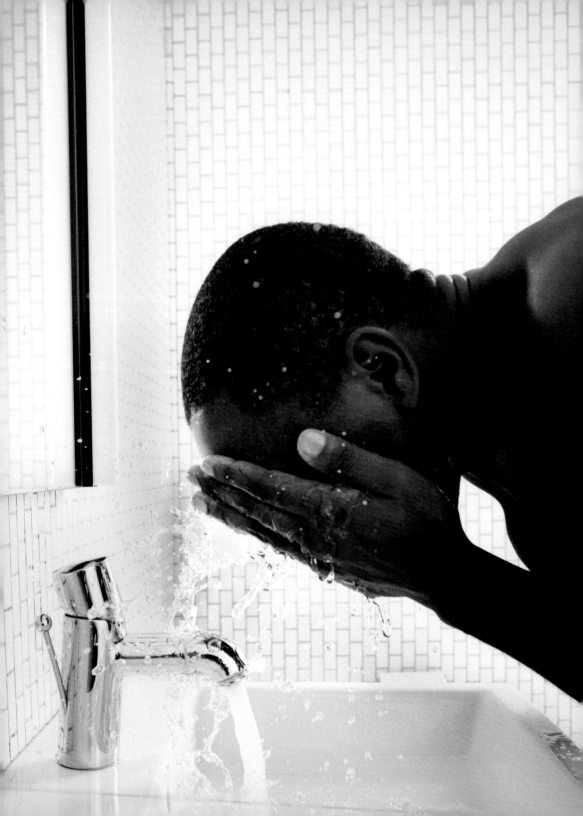

SKINCARE & GROOMING 101

So here it is, men: the essential elements that form the foundation of good grooming and skincare for every man, regardless of his style, age, or unique character (more on that later). If you read nothing else in this book, these basics will help ground you, build your confidence, and ensure you put your best face forward.

Our skin is an ever-evolving organ, and its state of being brings many factors into consideration. There's age, humidity, temperature, restfulness, pollution—the list goes on and on. While there is a lot to consider when taking care of it, the goal is simple: Find well-crafted products that don't force you to constantly switch up your routine. The right skin-care regimen should work with the chemistry of your body—not against it—and be able to handle whatever life throws at it.

YOUR FACE

Every day you must perform essential tasks for your face, without fail: **cleanse, moisturize, protect.** In that order. All three are required to keep the skin on your face balanced, looking healthy, and protected from the elements. Skip one (or all) of these steps and pores get clogged, blemishes may appear (or increase), oil production goes wild, and your skin will show signs of aging much sooner than it should. This doesn't have to be an elaborate ritual; at its simplest you can get away with one product for cleansing and another that will both moisturize and provide sun protection. You can handle two products, right? We will get into the specific products and detailed steps that work best in just a bit—and how to use them in the best way for you.

To start, though, choose a facial cleansing product with a bit of menthol and an exfoliant, and spend a little time washing your face. A two-minute lather-and-massage will reinvigorate your skin as it washes away the remains of the day. Rinse clean with warm (not hot) water, pat dry, and slather on the moisturizer. Every time. In my experience, even men who are committed to sun protection sometimes skip the step of moisturizing. But simply protecting against sun damage won't prevent your skin from looking old before its time. Wrinkles deepen over time, and adding a healthy dose of hydration keeps your skin plumped, making the wrinkles appear less pronounced. Choose a moisturizer that includes ingredients such as copper, calcium, and hyaluronic acid to improve elasticity.

Last, and most important, keep a trustworthy dermatologist in your contacts list. Whether dealing with minor skin issues or more serious conditions, a knowledgeable dermatologist is an absolute game-changer. See him or her once a year.

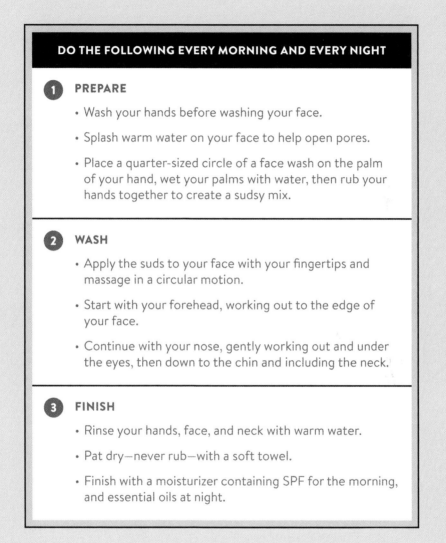

DO THE FOLLOWING EVERY MORNING AND EVERY NIGHT

1 PREPARE

- Wash your hands before washing your face.

- Splash warm water on your face to help open pores.

- Place a quarter-sized circle of a face wash on the palm of your hand, wet your palms with water, then rub your hands together to create a sudsy mix.

2 WASH

- Apply the suds to your face with your fingertips and massage in a circular motion.

- Start with your forehead, working out to the edge of your face.

- Continue with your nose, gently working out and under the eyes, then down to the chin and including the neck.

3 FINISH

- Rinse your hands, face, and neck with warm water.

- Pat dry—never rub—with a soft towel.

- Finish with a moisturizer containing SPF for the morning, and essential oils at night.

SHAVE LIKE YOU MEAN IT

Shaving isn't a slap'n'go effort, though many treat it that way. If you are going to take a sharpened blade to your face, you should do so with both care and intent. Few things can make a man look more polished than a close shave—think George Clooney or Jon Hamm as Don Draper—or more damaged, when things go wrong.

If you choose to shave with an electric razor, always start with a dry face and beard. Follow the manufacturer's specific instructions for the type of razor you have purchased, and clean the device after each use. Finish off your shave with an alcohol-free (or herbal) toner or an aftershave balm to soothe the skin.

—

TO MAKE SHAVING WITH A BLADE GO SMOOTHLY, FOLLOW THESE SIMPLE STEPS

1 PREPARE

- Shave only with a fresh, sharp blade.

- Before shaving prepare your beard by holding a steaming hot towel over the entire area to be shaved for three minutes. You can soak the towel in hot water or pop it in the microwave until it is just hot to the touch.

- Use a non-foaming shave cream rich in emollients. If you like, use a couple of drops of shave oil before the cream to help soften the beard and make shaving smoother.

2 SHAVE

- Using smooth, continuous strokes, draw the blade across your skin in the direction of hair growth, *not* against it. Never dig into the face or use short, choppy motions.

- Tighten delicate skin around the mouth or looser skin on the neck by pulling on it gently to help prevent nicking.

3 FINISH

- Rinse your face, removing all remnants of the shave cream.

- Pat the face dry with a soft towel.

- Finish with an alcohol-free or herbal toner, then apply your daily moisturizer with SPF.

FOCUS ON THE EYES

Think of your body as a plant. It requires the right amount of sunlight (a good source of Vitamin D) and hydration to look and feel its best.

Signs of fatigue and stress tend to show up first in the delicate skin around the eyes as dark circles, discoloration, or lines. The skin around your eyes is thinner than on the rest of your face and contains one-third fewer natural oils. There are a number of reasons dark circles occur, ranging from genetics to lack of sleep, but moisturizers and cover-up with Vitamin C will help brighten the area over time. An ice-cold washcloth held gently against the eyes can help reduce puffiness and dark circles, making bags under the eyes appear less pronounced. Use in the morning or before an evening out. Drink around eight glasses of water a day, get at least eight hours of sleep, and top yourself off with an eye cream before bed.

Pamper the eye area with a product specially formulated for the purpose, whether a serum, cream, or gel. It's different, and should be treated differently.

---

1 Use the tip of your ring finger to apply moisturizers or antiaging products under the eye. It has the most padding, and will be the easiest on delicate skin.

2 Apply by dabbing under each eye, from near your nose, outward toward your cheekbone.

3 Smooth and blend in any excess.

FACIAL HAIR

Man has had a tumultuous relationship with facial grooming. Whether mutton chops, Fu Manchus, or the chinstrap, every era seems to have a representative facial adornment—some more timeless than others. Fortunately, facial hair missteps are relatively quick and easy to fix, so there's no reason not to experiment. Beards are no longer limited to lumberjacks and pirates—these days, it seems like everyone is rocking one. With the right tools and techniques you can sport a 'stache or other facial flourish that makes the most of your features and presents the best version of yourself.

First, determine the volume that makes sense for your lifestyle. Do you perform in a band by the name of ZZ Top? If not, keep your beard trimmed and maintain it on a regular basis. Remember, a beard can add length or definition to the shape of your face, so choose a style with that in mind. Rounder faces can benefit from a squared-off beard shape and a bit of length at the chin. Narrower faces can be balanced with a fuller beard.

Fade your beard line smoothly into your neck. A sharp line is too severe—and calls extra attention to your chin(s). Use a trimmer to buzz from your Adam's apple to about two inches below your jawline.

Incorporate beard oil into your routine. It keeps beard hair looking bright and healthy, and makes it softer and easier to trim.

And when in doubt, find a photo of Sean Connery. Study it. He's your guy.

GET THE HEADLINE ON HAIR

It is often said that your hair is your most essential accessory, and nothing sends a stronger message about your sense of style than how you wear your hair. Whether long or short, a style that works for your personality, age, and profession is key to your comfort and confidence. A good cut establishes the shape; styling keeps it in place. You need to give thought to both.

Whatever you choose, find a look that's easy to maintain. Then treat it respectfully with high-quality products that nourish your hair and scalp. Products with coconut, avocado, or argan oils among their ingredients will give your hair a noticeable luster. Not sure if your hair is dry, normal, or oily? Ask your barber or stylist, who will certainly know. You can also ask your dermatologist.

If you are facing thinning hair, take it from me, there is no way to hide it, so deal with it instead. Toupees and comb-overs are for the birds—and you do not want anyone to see a nest on your head. On the other hand, a purposefully shaved head can be very attractive. A true man exudes confidence, even when he's not so sure about himself. (And if you do decide to embrace the bald, be sure to follow your daily dome shave with SPF protection on the scalp.)

I've always found that a head of gray hair can look classic and distinguished. If you're only beginning to gray, a careful touch of color can take years off, quickly. Too much color, though, only confirms the situation and the effort to cover it. Avoid fashion-inspired dye jobs. Hair grays because it loses pigment, which will inevitably change the texture of your hair. It becomes coarser, too. Nothing makes a man look older than a dated cut. So if you're going gray, go for something more modern, but not necessarily the style sported by the youngest person you know. You will not only look more up-to-date you may well feel younger, too.

FOR GREAT HAIR:

1 Admit that "not caring about it" isn't the right approach. Even relaxed guys have a style they make their own.

2 Update your style with the help of a professional stylist and maintain it at least every six weeks. See a barber every other week for trims and touch-ups.

3 Style your hair daily; without a little help from a styling gel or paste, the best cut in the world won't hold its shape.

BELOW THE BELT

As for the rest of your body, that often comes down to personal preference. Don't go overboard with the manscaping. Body hair should look natural, but not out of control. Keep forearms and legs as they are, and keep the chest region in line with your own personal tastes. Remember: There's a reason why so many people fawn over Hugh Jackman. When trimming, always trim with the natural growth of the hair, and move slowly to avoid overtrimming or too close a pruning. If you're going for a Channing Tatum look, use a transparent shave gel to better see what you are doing, and shave in the direction of the hair growth. If you're really committed to a smooth, hairless chest, waxing or laser treatments give more permanent results. Whichever method you choose, proceed with caution around any sensitive areas.

Laser treatments are a good option for trouble areas that you are tired of dealing with—the shoulders, for example. As for back hair, it's a part of life that many are uncomfortable with. If you decide to deal with it, it will require the help of a professional or a friend. If you are especially hirsute and comfortable with it, then rock what you have and be proud of your follicular abundance. Remember, there's nothing more attractive than confidence.

When it comes to trimming in the trousers, an electric trimmer is best for achieving a uniform look. Again, go with the growth pattern and move slowly.

FOR BODY HAIR:

1 Maintain it as carefully as the hair on your head or on your face, if you have any.

2 Choose the style that you feel the most confident with. Forget magazine trends and do what is right for you in this especially personal area.

3 Always go with the growth of the hair, whether trimming or shaving—and that's true both above and below the belt. When trimming, remember you can always make a second pass if needed. Don't take off too much.

LEND ME A HAND—AND A FOOT

Use a hand salve at least once a week to keep hands hydrated and to help prevent cracking. In dry weather, or if you are doing a lot of manual labor, moisturize your hands daily to counteract the drying effects of frequent washing or harsh chemicals.

And don't neglect your feet. Treat your feet well. As needed, use a scrub brush or pumice stone to keep rough skin in check, and a good heel salve to keep your feet as healthy as possible.

It's also a good idea to turn yourself over to a pro every now and then. The ladies may have claimed the nail spa as a female-only domain, but hey, you can't spell manicure without "man," right? Put your foot down—and get a pedicure. Stop in for a moisturizing hand massage, and ask the technician to clean up your hangnails and cuticles, but pass on the polish. A quick buff is all you need—and it feels great.

FOR HEALTHY HANDS AND FEET:

1 Remember that moisturizers, salves, and balms help keep hands soft and younger looking. They are visible to all, and as part of a handshake, play a key role in making your first impression.

2 Treat your feet especially well if for no other reason than they take the entire weight of your life journey. Use a scrub brush on them daily to keep down calluses and to help prevent odor.

3 Trust professionals to help you, just as you do when choosing a stylist for you hair or a dermatologist for your skin.

Take these basics to heart.
Use them with confidence, and
incorporate all that apply into a
deliberate daily grooming program.
When you take a more intentional
approach to your routine, you'll
feel the difference both inside and
out. It may seem a bit fussy at first,
but even a few small tweaks and
bit of additional effort will pay
dividends almost immediately,
giving you a subtle but definite air
of sophistication and confidence
that others will pick up on. Isn't
that worth a few extra minutes in
the morning and evening?

GETTING THE JOB
DONE RIGHT

2

WHAT EVERY MAN SHOULD HAVE, KNOW, AND USE

Even if your father never sat you down and taught you how to shave, he probably did tell you at one time or another, "To do the job right, you need the right tool for the job." When it comes to grooming, that advice is as spot-on as it is in the workshop. If you've always been a soap-and-water and lip balm kind of guy, now's the time to expand your horizons . . . just a bit. I'm not here to talk you into a complicated, ten-part, product-heavy ritual. But there are reasons that there are different products for moisturizing different parts of the body, and why the cleanser you use on your hands after working in the garden or garage shouldn't be the same one you use on your face. It makes you informed, not narcissistic, to know your way around a few basic products. What follows will help you make the best choices for your needs when you shop and ensure you have the basics covered, both at home and away.

CHOOSE PRODUCTS WITH CONFIDENCE

If it seems like there are a million products out there, most touting special benefits, you're not wrong. But not every product will be right for you and your skin. So let's cut through the clutter and start with finding what will work for you.

SOME BASIC KNOWLEDGE BEFORE YOU SHOP

- Do some research before you head into the store, just as you would when buying any new product. Poll your friends and look online, actually *reading* the customer reviews.

- You want products that say what they do and do what they say. Experiment and find the ones you trust.

- You don't have to spend a fortune on good skincare and grooming. More affordable products can often work well, but don't skimp on price at the expense of the right ingredients or what works best for you.

HAIR

- When it comes to shampoo and conditioner, it's simple: Identify your hair type and buy formulations meant for that type.

- For styling products, look for detailed descriptors of functional benefits (amount of hold or flexibility, for example). Good products tell you what they do. Play with the testers whenever available to determine what works for you.

SKIN

- The best moisturizers are formulated with gentle ingredients that have been found to be the most compatible with the skin's own natural oils. Use what you know about your skin type, environment, and personal preference to choose the best formula for you.

- Sunscreen with an SPF of at least 50 is nonnegotiable. It's a known fact that sun ages the skin, so you have to protect yourself. Look for a formula with antioxidant Vitamin E or goji berry to provide increased protection from free-radical damage. You want a formula that feels good and works with your routine so you continue to use it daily.

- If you spend a great deal of time indoors, consider a self-tanner or bronzer to give a healthy glow to skin. Be sure to read instructions carefully.

EYES AND EYEBROWS

- Pick up a moisturizer specifically formulated for the eye area, where the skin is thinner.

- Get a pair of good-quality tweezers, not bargain-basement options. You'll drive yourself crazy trying to grab at that one hair with dull tweezers.

LIPS

- Cracked lips are never attractive, so find something that's portable and won't melt in your pocket. Pots of salve may have a nicer consistency than lip balm in a tube, but for sanitary reasons you don't want to be dipping your finger into a jar repeatedly.

BODY AND BODY HAIR

- Look for products that absorb easily into your skin type, rather than sit on top of it or feel gummy to you. The skin on your body is thicker than the skin on your face, so test what feels right.

- Get a body trimmer if you intend to groom. Do not use basic barber or hair clippers for this job.

HANDS AND NAILS

- Whenever testers are available, use them. It is important that you like the feel of the products on your hands, or you'll end up not using them at all. Purchase the one that feels lightest and least greasy on your skin.

BEARD

- Facial hair is different from the hair on your head or body; it is thicker and coarser. Don't confuse shave oils for beard oils. The first are used to prepare the skin for shaving, the second to keep facial hair looking great. Buy both.

- Get an adjustable beard trimmer. Do not use basic barber or hair clippers for this task.

KEY INGREDIENTS & THEIR BENEFITS

It pays to read labels and have a basic understanding of which active ingredients will be most beneficial to your skin type. This will ensure you are not wasting money on benefits you don't want or need or, even worse, aggravate the situation. Using products with the appropriate ingredients for your skin and hair condition will give you the results you're looking for.

HAIR

- Coconut oil moisturizes.
- Avocado oil helps replace natural oils.
- Argan oil improves texture.

EYES

- Vitamin C helps brighten discoloration and circles.
- Caffeine reduces puffiness.

LIPS

- Shea butter protects skin from dehydration and improves the skin's appearance.
- Vitamin E prevents free radicals, and soothes and moisturizes lips.
- Aloe vera helps soften lips.

BODY

- Aloe vera softens and soothes skin.

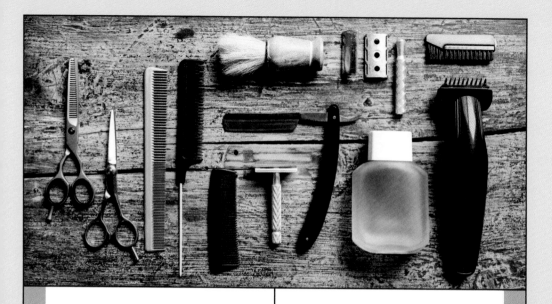

SKIN

- Copper and calcium help prevent aging skin.

- Squalane restores skin's natural moisture balance.

- Clay draws out imperfections.

- Calendula and centella soothe skin.

- Vitamin C improves the appearance of aging skin.

- Vitamin E protects against free radicals to prevent aging skin.

- Menthol feels cool and refreshing on the skin.

- Caffeine reduces puffiness.

- Sunscreen with an SPF of at least 50, plus goji berry, protects skin.

BEARD

- Eucalyptus extract penetrates the hair and invigorates skin under the beard.

- Rosemary oil provides antioxidant properties.

- Spearmint refreshes the beard and senses.

HANDS & NAILS

- Avocado oil helps replace skin's natural moisture.

- Sesame oil softens dry, cracked, or chapped hands.

KNOW THE TERMINOLOGY NEEDED TO BUY WHAT'S BEST FOR YOU

There is no shortage of terminology, descriptors, and product names. It's enough to make many men give up on skincare and grooming entirely. Taking care of yourself starts with taking time to learn a bit about what will actually work for your needs. And you should know a cream from a gel from a serum. Here's the lowdown:

HAIRCARE

There are so many haircare products on the market, it can be very confusing which to choose. Part of it comes down to hair type and personal preference. A little experimentation and advice from your barber or stylist can help you determine which is right for you.

. . . .

Cream: Hair creams smooth and protect hair. Best for those with a relaxed, casual hairstyle, creams are also perfect for de-frizzing coarse hair or, when used sparingly, adding texture to slightly thinning hair.

Gel: Gels are available in both light- and firm-hold formulas. As a general rule, the finer your hair, the lighter the gel you should use. Some gels can become flaky once they set, so test-drive your gel before a special event.

. . . .

Pomade: Wax- or water-based pomades give hair shine and luster. If you're going for a slick, well-groomed hairstyle, using a pomade is your best option. You can change the style by altering the amount of pomade you use and whether you apply it to wet or dry hair. When applied to wet hair, pomade will give less hold with more shine; when applied to dry hair, pomade will give more hold with less shine. Today's formulas are less sticky than the products your grandfather used.

. . . .

Waxes and Pastes: Waxes will truly "hold" a hairstyle and are usually a better choice than pomade for those with oily hair. Wax doesn't remain malleable in the hair, but today's formulas are water soluble, so you can easily wash it out in your next shower. Pastes allow you to mold your hair into the style of your choice without making it stiff or crunchy. They also add strength and vitality to hair.

FACIAL SKINCARE

Your face makes the first impression. Take care of it. Talk to your skincare specialist to learn more about your skin type and the skincare regimen best suited for your face and specific needs.

. . . .

Cleanser: High-quality facial cleansers are low-lathering or non-foaming to help maintain the skin's natural oil base. They remove dirt, debris, and oily residue from the skin.

. . . .

Exfoliant: These facial scrubs slough off dead skin cells that build up on the surface of the skin and cause dullness. Regular exfoliation (one to three times a week) leaves the skin feeling silky-soft and primed for moisturizing. Those with acne-prone or very sensitive skin should not use facial scrubs, to avoid irritation or redness.

. . . .

Toner: Facial toners remove excess dirt, debris, or cleanser residue. Use a few drops on a sterile cotton pad or as an after-shave splash to help soothe razor discomfort after shaving.

. . . .

Serum: Serums are thinner than moisturizing lotions and are typically dispensed from a pump or dropper. Serums are formulated with ingredients that target a particular skincare concern and are designed to penetrate the skin more deeply than a moisturizer.

. . . .

Moisturizer: Facial moisturizers retain and replenish moisture loss in facial skin. Moisturizers are sold in a variety of textures and sun protection factors to suit most skin types and to accommodate different lifestyles. Whether you use a lighter or heavier moisturizer will depend on your skin type, environmental conditions, and personal preferences.

Lotion: Lotions come in the lightest-weight formulas, and are easily absorbed and nongreasy. Those with oily skin generally prefer lotions due to their lightweight feel on the skin and tendency not to clog pores. Those with oil throughout the face, especially on the chin, nose, and forehead, may experience blemishes and/or breakouts.

Cream: Creams are light-textured, hydrating, and soothing. Creams are right for all skin types but those whose skin types are normal to oily (*slight shine in the T-zone—forehead, nose, and chin*), normal (*skin feels comfortable*), and normal to dry (*comfortable T-zone, taut cheeks, may experience flakiness*) generally prefer them.

Balm: Balms have a thick, rich, buttery texture and are deeply nourishing. Balms are perfect for dry to very dry skin types that often feel parched, taut, or tight, and may experience flakiness.

Eye Cream/Eye Serum: Eye creams and serums help address dryness and aging in the delicate eye area. Using an eye cream or serum consistently, along with sunscreen and sunglasses, can significantly protect the eye-area skin and maintain its appearance over time.

. . . .

Masques: Masques address facial imbalances such as clogged pores or dryness. If the imbalance is isolated, it's best to use the masques in those specific zones, otherwise they can be used on the entire face (always avoiding the eyes or other sensitive areas). For best results, apply one to three times per week.

SHAVING AND BEARD CARE

Every man has his own preference for his shaving and beard-care rituals. Whatever yours is, there are a few basics that will make you happier with the results.

. . . .

Shave Cream: For those who use manual razors, shave cream provides the closest and most comfortable shave. Look for formulas containing aloe, squalane, or palm oil, which contribute to a creamy consistency that helps shield the face from razor impact and irritation. However, a thick layer applied to a wet face can ultimately clog your razor. To avoid this, apply a thin layer over damp, not wet, skin.

Post-Shave Treatment: These specially formulated tonics, gels, and razor-bump relief lotions calm, soothe, nourish, and invigorate a closely shaven face, leaving skin soft, smooth, and comfortable.

. . . .

Beard Oil: Applied before shaving—preferably in the shower, where the steamy heat can help the oils penetrate more deeply—beard oil softens facial hair, making it easier to shave off, helping prevent razor burn. They are formulated with natural oils that help protect, comfort, and moisturize skin, and are particularly recommended for men with sensitive skin or a tough beard, or a tendency toward ingrown hairs or razor burn.

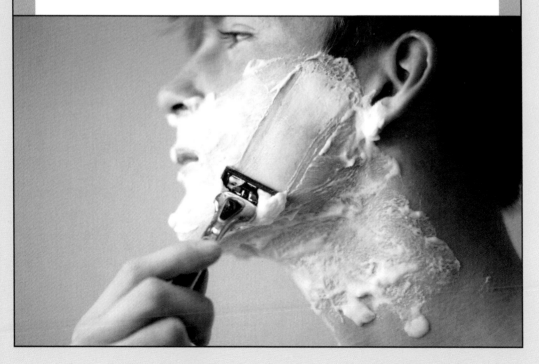

WHAT YOU NEED AND WHERE

IN YOUR SHOWER AT HOME

☐ **SHAMPOO AND CONDITIONER**
Keeping hair properly cleansed and hydrated is key to a great hairstyle.

☐ **FACE AND BODY CLEANSER**
You're in the shower to get clean, so do it. Regular bar soap can dry your skin, unless it contains moisturizing ingredients and oils.

☐ **EXFOLIATOR**
Exfoliating ensures that your products penetrate deeper and work better.

IN YOUR DOPP KIT OR GYM BAG

☐ **EYE CREAM**
Eye products are essential while traveling because they help battle the signs of lack of sleep or jet lag.

☐ **ALL-IN-ONE FACE/BODY/HAIR WASH**
A formula that does triple duty is great for when away from home.

☐ **MOISTURIZER WITH AN SPF OF AT LEAST 50**
A good double duty product to streamline what needs doing.

☐ **BLOTTING PAPERS**
These are an easy way to pat away excess oil when you can't stop to wash and re-moisturize.

IN YOUR MEDICINE CABINET & BATHROOM

☐ **FACIAL CLEANSER**
To remove debris and excess oil gently.

☐ **TONER**
If you have oily skin, toner is a crucial step to managing it.

☐ **EYE CREAM**
The first signs of aging appear around the eyes, so battle it.

☐ **MOISTURIZER**
Hydrated skin is vitally important in face and body care.

☐ **SUNSCREEN**
One with an SPF of at least 50 is a must for faces (and bald heads), to prevent sun damage, wrinkling, and skin cancer.

☐ **CONCEALER**
There are some imperfections that great skincare can't fix immediately; use concealer to hide these.

☐ **TRIMMER WITH MULTIPLE CLIP SETTINGS**
Start at the highest clip (e.g., 3) and work your way down when trimming.

☐ **SHARP BEARD AND MUSTACHE SCISSORS, AND BEARD BRUSH**
Use for finer touch-ups and stray hairs.

☐ **BEARD OIL OR CONDITIONER**
To keep facial hair from getting wiry.

☐ **SHAVING OIL, CREAM, AND RAZOR**
To prepare skin for a smoother, nick-free shave that foams just can't provide.

QUESTIONS
FROM REAL LIFE

3

KEY ANSWERS & USEFUL TIPS
FROM SOMEONE ON THE FRONT LINE

I never know when I will get a grooming question from someone: it could be via e-mail from a customer I've met, or a text from a friend getting ready for an event, or from a stranger who recognizes me while I'm working out at the gym. I'm always glad to get them, and just as surprised by how similar many of their questions are. It all leads me to assume that today's man has a real need for real information. I've addressed the basics in the previous section; now we can apply those fundamentals to the questions I get asked most often.

You may find the questions here are similar to your own, unexpected and enlightening, or quite basic. Wherever you find yourself on this spectrum, I'm guessing there are still times you find yourself needing some direction on what to do, how frequently it should be done, and who to trust when you need to turn to a professional. If so, don't feel bad. With very few exceptions most of the men I encounter would love to know how to freshen up their looks and simply don't know where to start or who to ask. That's where I come in.

By far the most common subject I am asked about is hair. Hardly surprising, as hair (or a lack thereof) is associated with vanity, with masculinity, with aging. And it's not just the hair on top of their heads—or on their heads at all, for that matter—that's got men looking for guidance. One of the things that makes me happiest is the trust people put in me. It is a real honor when men feel they can "ask me anything"—and they do. The truth is, these "awkward" questions also need to be addressed, and this book is the safest place to take them on. Manscaping? Man makeup? Body odor? I've heard it all, and I'll give you the straight scoop. Here are a few of the queries that have come my way the most often:

I shave every day, but don't really know the "right way." What's the best technique?

First you need to determine whether you want to use an electric shaver, a disposable "safety" razor, or an old-school straight razor like the ones barbers use (which may look cool but have no protective features). Choice is a matter of personal comfort. Generally, people with sensitive skin or light beards gravitate toward electric razors because they're gentler on the skin. Those with heavier beards tend to prefer a manual razor. An electric razor is easier in that you can use it anytime, and there's minor prep required. If you use a traditional razor, as I do, the process of shaving takes a little more time and prep. I prefer to shave in the morning before I shower. First, I wet a washcloth with the hottest water I can stand and hold it against any area I plan to shave. This stands the hair up and softens it as well, so you can get the closest possible shave. I use a shave cream rather than a foam because foams (or a

HERE IS WHAT TO DO WHEN SHAVING

1 PREPARE   Hold a hot, wet washcloth against the area
to be shaved until the towel just starts to cool.
About 2 to 3 minutes, generally.

2 LUBRICATE   Use light shave oil or shave cream to ensure smooth
movement of the razor.

3 EXECUTE   Shave in the direction of hair growth, **not** against it,
using long, smooth motions.

4 FINISH   Soothe the face with an herbal toner and light
moisturizer. If you have a beard, condition it with
2 to 3 drops of beard oil.

Shave in the direction
of hair growth, **not**
against it, using long,
smooth motions.

too-thick layer of cream) may create air pockets that can cause you to nick yourself. Shave creams are also mistake-proof—if you've shaved away the cream, you can be sure you haven't missed any spots. If you have facial hair, it's good to use a clear product (such as an oil) that provides lubrication but doesn't cover up your hair so you don't accidentally take off a sideburn or half your mustache. I finish by washing my face with a bit of cleanser on the same washcloth. It's important to remove any residue from the shaving cream and cleanser.

What can I do about my wrinkles?

Focus on hydration. Wrinkles are visible because the grooves in your skin create areas of dark and light, and they deepen over time. Any topical product plumps those grooves and therefore reduces the appearance of the lines. The more often you moisturize, the better results you will see over time. Think of it this way: If you never treat your car's dashboard, over time the sun will make it cracked and dull. The skin on your face reacts to the sun and elements in a similar way. Moisturizers condition the face and help it retain essential oils so lines don't occur as early or severely. Drinking plenty of water to stay hydrated helps, too. The other key piece is protecting your face from the sun. If you're not using sunscreen, you're trying to fill a bucket with a hole in the bottom.

If you already follow a solid moisturizer and sunscreen routine, and you're still seeing lines appear or worsen, use products with age-fighting ingredients like copper, calcium, and hyaluronic acid to improve skin's elasticity, and squalane to keep your skin hydrated.

THIS IS WHAT TO DO FOR WRINKLES

1 PREPARE — Ensure wrinkled areas are clean.

2 APPLY — Use a light moisturizer with SPF during the day. At night, apply an essential oils serum, then a cream moisturizer.

3 EXECUTE — Apply moisturizer all over your face, including the neck area, which will wrinkle more over time.

4 FINISH — Drink a large glass of water after you moisturize; there is no point in trying to keep moisture in if there isn't enough hydration internally.

If I moisturize, do I need a separate eye cream?

Because the skin in the under-eye area is one-third as thick as other facial skin, and contains one-third fewer oil glands, it's the first place signs of aging occur, making eye cream a crucial component of your daily moisturizing routine. It's important to use products specifically formulated for the eye area because you want ingredients that won't migrate into the eye and cause irritation. So, yes, you really do need two moisturizing products for your face.

THIS IS WHAT TO DO FOR THE EYES

1 PREPARE   Gently wash your face, including around the eye area, and pat dry.

2 APPLY   Place a small amount (about the size of a pea or less) of your chosen product under each eye, just above the cheekbone and away from the lash line.

3 EXECUTE   Gently dab the product onto the entire under-eye area with the tip of your ring finger—it has the most padding and will be the gentlest—moving from the center of your face toward the hairline. Be sure to apply product all the way up through the area where "crow's feet" can appear.

4 FINISH   Smooth out any excess and blend it in.

The tip of your ring finger has the most padding and will be the gentlest.

Move from the center of your face toward the hairline.

Apply product all the way up through the area where "crow's feet" can appear.

Barber or stylist?

Both. A stylist is someone you can work with to create a look that's right for your face, age, and profession. A barber is great for touching up an existing cut inexpensively. You should have one of each, and focus on communication to build trust. Don't be led to a radical new look by a stylist unless you really want to shake things up. At the same time, don't be afraid to ask if it's time to update your look, and don't let a barber buzz off all your hair if you just want the ear and neck areas cleaned up.

> Remember: A stylist will create a look that is right for your face, age, and profession; a barber will maintain the lines and keep it tidy in between visits to the stylist. Communication is key with both.

How often do you get a haircut?

Every three weeks—whether that's going to the barber for a cleanup, or my stylist for a rework. It shouldn't be left up to "when there is time," or when it's obviously been too long. I get touch-ups as needed, depending on the style of my cut. The shorter and cleaner the cut, the more important touch-ups are, and the more frequent they need to be. Any overgrowth near the ears or neck can quickly look sloppy. Make grooming a scheduled part of your good habits, and you will look your best all the time. An added bonus: If you have a beard, your barber can help keep it in shape, too.

What should I use in my hair?

It depends on what your hair is like and how comfortable you are using styling products. But unless you are sporting a brush cut or have opted to shave it all off, odds are your hair will look and behave better with a little product on board. The cut is the shape and length of hair; the style is how you work those features to look your best. In general, longer cuts are better styled smoothly or loosely, and shorter cuts look best when styled with a stronger-holding product.

I have medium-thick hair, so I begin by using a product that will moisturize and protect it, and finish with a pomade or shaping paste to hold the style in place. If you have longer, curlier, or very thin hair, you might want to experiment with various products to see what works best for you. Don't be afraid to explore both cut and styling, and ask your stylist which products will keep things looking sharp.

What are your thoughts on coloring hair? If I do color my hair, should I color my beard, too? My eyebrows? Should they match?

Hair color is an interesting topic for men. I do believe that if you color your hair, your facial hair should match. If you have a little bit of gray, covering it up will remove years from your look. Off-the-shelf products can be effective for covering gray if you are less than 25% gray on your head or beard, but let professionals do anything involving a lot of color or sensitive areas, especially your eyebrows. Because that area is so sensitive, coloring them yourself could go very wrong very quickly—including chemical damage, loss of hair, and ending up way too dark and looking clownish.

What about seasonal haircuts?

If you're following the trend of a seasonal haircut—super short for summer, for example—I strongly suggest you go to a professional and bring a photo. Not all haircuts are suited for all hair types, face shapes, or ages. It's crucial to find the right professional to both assess the best styles for your hair and be honest about which are appropriate for you.

> **Remember:** Great style isn't about being trendy; it's about what works best for you and makes you look and feel most confident.

Some men have questions that go beyond the basics, wondering about more "technical" things that others ignore. There is no requirement to wear fragrance, pluck eyebrows, or address problem areas, but if you choose to, here's how to go about it correctly.

How do you feel about men and fragrance?

Rule number 1 (and 2 and 3) is don't use too much if you do wear fragrance. You never want your fragrance to enter the room before you do. I spray once on both sides of the neck and both wrists. Never chafe your wrists together after; it crushes the notes and muddles the fragrance.

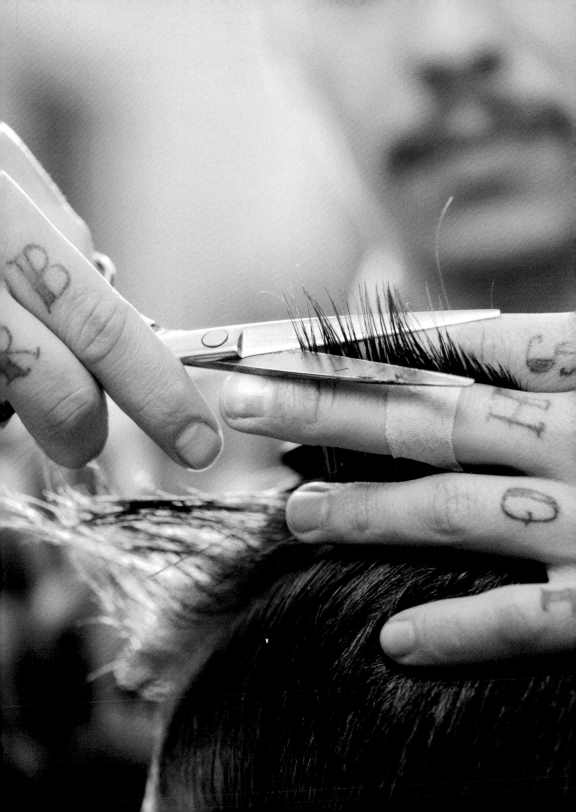

Choose lighter scents for summer and more complex ones for winter. A signature scent can be a cornerstone of how you present yourself. Scent also triggers memory, so sticking with just a couple will help establish comfort and bonding of all sorts.

Soaps, lotions, and deodorants also add to your scent, so be cautious of too many scents together becoming overpowering or conflicting with each other.

Do I need to pluck my brows?

Let's just assume you do—almost everyone needs to clean up their brows. The goal is not to draw attention to the brows, but instead to the eyes. Nothing frames your eyes (and face) better than a shapely eyebrow, and brows that are too bushy, or heavy, or scraggly can make you look tired, messy, or just unkempt. The secret to plucking is never to look plucked. Groom the brows by cleaning up the hairs between and under them, but not above. You don't want to change their natural shape. To get the right shape, go to a professional for the first attempt. Then, clean up in key areas and remove obvious strays, but don't work against the existing shape of the brow. You can also use a brow trimmer with a guard to keep things in check, or a small brush to smooth them out. Tend to your brows every three weeks.

Why do I get ingrown hairs? How can I treat or prevent them?

Ingrown hairs occur when new hair growth doesn't effectively break through the skin's surface and grows back in toward the follicle, causing a bump or whitehead to form under the skin.

Regular exfoliation will prevent your pores from getting clogged; use very warm water when you cleanse your face to help keep the pores clean and open. If you're prone to ingrown hairs, a razor bump relief product is a great preventative measure.

> **Ingrown outtake:** Exfoliation should prevent ingrown hairs over time. But if there is a hair growing under the skin like a splinter, or back on itself into the follicle, see a dermatologist to take care of it. Ingrown hairs can resolve themselves on their own, but often not before becoming irritated or inflamed. Don't dig at your face with tweezers or other instruments; you can scar your skin and risk infection, causing further damage.

Manscaping. How much is too much?

You want to look natural but not out of control. I'm of the belief that arms and legs should be natural. If I had a lot of body hair all over, I wouldn't necessarily wax my chest, but I would probably wax my back. But, as I noted earlier, if you are especially hirsute, you should really think about whether you can learn to feel attractive and confident exactly as you are, or with minor tweaks. Consider getting laser treatments on trouble areas that you're sick of shaving or waxing all the time, like the tops of your shoulders or above the tailbone. Then leave the rest as is.

Whether you opt for a lot of or a little body hair maintenance, never manscape against the natural growth pattern of your body hair. Doing so will leave you looking patchy and uneven. Start with electric clippers on their middle setting, and work from the top of your chest downward. Use a brush to remove clipped hair and see the results. Repeat on a lower trimmer setting if necessary. Go slowly and make several passes to ensure you don't end up unexpectedly shorn like a sheep, unless that's the look you're going for. Address the areas below the waist last, to get a smooth transition in grooming.

Makeup? Really?

Makeup can both enhance and camouflage. A bit of self-tanning lotion or bronzer can help you look healthier after too much time indoors. If you have a pimple or hereditary dark circles, concealer can become your best friend, taking years off your face and quickly hiding something you don't want the world to see.

> **Remember:** If you do decide to use some form of makeup—bronzers or cover-up—the ultimate goal is to match and enhance your skin tone, not completely mask it. Under-eye concealer shouldn't be used for complete "white out" conditions, as it will look too obvious. Cover a blemish to reduce the redness, not hide the offender entirely, as that will tend to emphasize the product as much as the blemish itself. If you are appearing on television or in a video shoot, leave any other type of color to professionals, who will ensure you look natural.

What's the best approach to keeping a great smile?

Diligent, twice-daily brushing, flossing, and mouthwash are essential. And seeing your dentist no less than twice a year is a must. For crooked teeth, adult orthodontia is a temporary inconvenience for a long-lasting result. There are many treatments today that can give you invisible braces, and straighten your teeth faster than ever. It is possible to professionally whiten yellow teeth for a movie-star smile, but in the meantime, limit coffee and red wine, which can stain teeth.

If your budget is tight, every name brand toothpaste has an over-the-counter, daily-use treatment that will get your teeth looking their whitest. Carry mints and drink mint tea to keep breath fresh—and limit your intake of garlic and onion.

I seem to have perpetual body odor. Is there any hope for me?

This can be hereditary, or it can be due to your diet. There are soaps and cleansers formulated to help with this problem. Showering regularly and properly is important, so make it a priority. Give particular attention to "where parts meet"—armpits, crotch, between toes. This is where bacteria, the cause of body odors, can grow and linger. Fragrance and deodorants can help, but are absolutely not standalone solutions. You want to prevent the odors, not cover them up.

For starters, ensure your soap or shower gel has deodorizing properties. And watch what you eat; believe it or not, a diet heavy in spices, garlic, red meat, asparagus, or beer can add to body odor. Limit these foods to limit the issue—and drink lots of water every day to reduce concentrated odors after meals.

I sweat like a pig. What should I do about it?

If you sweat a lot, you need a strong antiperspirant and good hygiene. It's that simple. Plan on more than one shower each day, and keep a fresh shirt in both your office and your car. One tried-and-true solution is to wear a light cotton T-shirt under your dress shirt to absorb excess sweat. You may also want to speak with your dermatologist about the issue.

> **Remember:** Sweat may be unsightly and unpleasant, but it is also a sign that your body is using a lot of its water for cooling down or stress management. Be sure you replenish often to stay hydrated. To protect skin when outdoors, use a water-resistant or sweat-resistant moisturizer with an SPF of no less than 50.

I can't seem to control my acne. What's best?

First, make sure you're not addressing the problem too aggressively, as that can aggravate the situation. Keep your face clean but don't dry it out, which can happen if you are aggressively applying astringents or alcohol-based products. While it may seem counterintuitive, the strategic use of products with essential oils can actually reduce over-production of natural skin oils, and help balance your complexion over-all. You also want to look for products that will calm redness so the acne doesn't look inflamed.

Your skin is as unique as you are. Know and understand your skin type. See a skincare expert to help you determine your skin type, understand what you need to treat it, and follow the basics: cleanse, moisturize, protect. When the skin reaches a more natural state, a dermatologist can help address any medical issues. Most important, make sure to be well groomed in all other regards; it will deflect attention from the things you don't want people to focus on.

What about acne on my back?

Skincare doesn't stop with your face. You need to pay attention to *all* the skin on your body, including your back. Cleansing properly is critical. You have to wash your back actively, not just let water run down it in the shower. Gentle exfoliation with an exfoliating brush is also important—but gentle is key. If you have active acne, hard scrubbing will irritate it. Keeping pores clean and the skin properly moisturized will help stop acne over time.

Is it okay to shave my legs?

Unless you are an Olympic swimmer looking to also shave milliseconds off your 100-meter splits, don't do it. Shaved arms and legs never look natural, so avoid any temptation to find out.

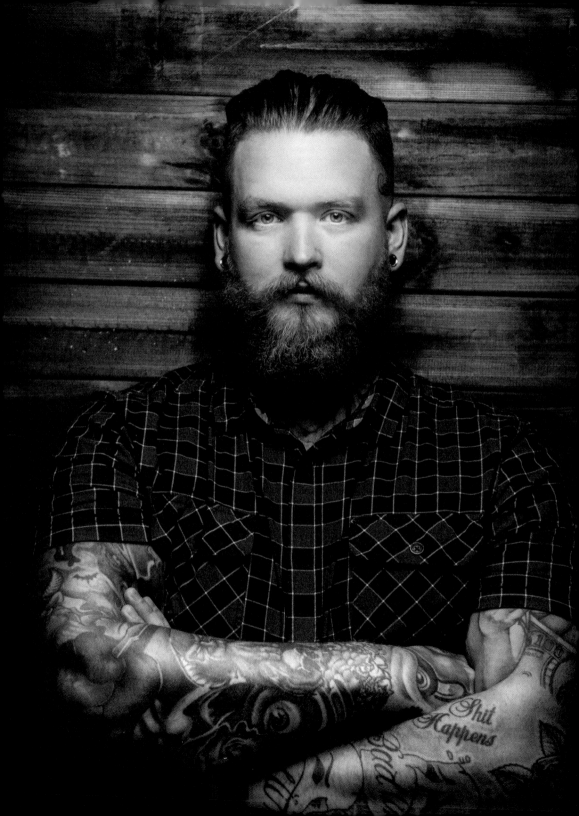

PART II

REAL MEN IN THEIR REAL WORLDS

THE MODERN GENTLEMAN

4

WHAT IT TAKES TO BE
POLISHED & ON POINT TODAY

Ask anybody. When describing you, the first word that comes to mind would be *polished*. Everything about you is refined: the way you dress, interact with others, present your opinions, work, live, care for yourself. Some may consider your gentlemanly manners a bit old school, and they aren't entirely wrong. You like to think of yourself as a classic—with a modern twist.

You knew early on that you could command attention. Whether in the boardroom or the living room you exude a sense of ease and control, something that makes people gravitate to you. This ability to draw people in has served you well as you traveled the world in pursuit of career and life interests. Your worldly charm is both refreshing and disarming, though you aren't above a good raunchy joke or occasional prank. In a tuxedo at a formal function or in jeans and a cashmere hoodie just kicking back with friends, it's clear you are comfortable in your own skin.

Impeccable timing is one of your key traits, and it gives your life and actions a clear sense of purpose. You believe in handwritten letters and thank-you notes, but understand that there are times when a quick e-mail or text are just as appropriate; nothing wrong with progress as long as form and function are matched perfectly to achieve a striking result. The same is true in social situations. Your quick mind and easy sense of humor have helped you diffuse many awkward moments. The more uncomfortable the situation, the more Zen you become, and your unflappable demeanor puts others at ease.

You've been brought up with a strong sense of ethics, and still take your direction from the strong moral compass instilled in you by your parents. Giving voice to those who don't have one and standing up for what you know to be right, even when unpopular, are values you embrace and live by. That family connection also keeps you grounded and serves as a reality check. Let's face it, a man cannot log tens of thousands of miles in airplanes every year and then tell others they should abandon their SUVs for a hybrid without looking false.

You travel and work. A lot. Your headspace is rarely less than maxed, but you will never let down a friend in need, forget a dear colleague's birthday, or show up empty-handed to a dinner party. It's not for show; it's in your DNA. You cannot help but pay attention to even small details.

Consequently you are meticulous in your approach to life and career. You know that to master your craft takes endless practice and an ongoing willingness to learn. You will never be done honing your skills, your mind, or your body; it's what keeps you engaged, energized, and at the top of your field.

You are a man of habits and rituals—*une bête d'habitude*—and your highly refined tastes require that you keep highly refined company. Your Rolodex is a who's who: best men's tailor in Hong Kong; most romantic restaurant in Rome; perfect spa in the Swiss Alps; latest design wunderkind in Stockholm. Check, check, check, and check. It's not that you won't explore and add new ideas to your repertoire. However, your threshold is as high as the one you set for yourself: make it impeccable, make it seem effortless. Nobody ought to know how much work and thought goes into your way of life—the real payoff is that people think it comes to you naturally.

When it comes to grooming, you cultivate your appearance as thoughtfully as you do every other aspect of your life. After all, your body and fine mind are the keys to your success. The right diet, a balanced workout regimen—from meditation to swimming—and carefully chosen grooming rituals keep you polished no matter where you are in the world. Many of your rituals have been informed by your travels and your study of other cultures. You've noted, for example, that Italian men care about their appearance as much as their female counterparts. Though you might find them a bit over the top sometimes, you enjoy their exuberance and panache when it comes to fashion. Asia, on the other hand, is a case study in how to work hard and play harder. Nobody does spa culture better. And you cherry-pick from each of these traditions to create your own code of conduct for grooming and self-care.

Above all, you always need something to look forward to, to keep life from becoming predictable. After all, there is nothing that gets your blood flowing like taking the stage to announce: "Ladies and gentlemen, may I have your attention?" **Once you have it, what do you do with it? The first thing: Do your part to look the part.**

STYLE NOTES FOR THE POLISHED GENTLEMAN

- Actively mitigate the effects of frequent travel and long work hours—looking polished takes extra effort.

- Project a refined image even when dressed casually— the gentleman knows every impression matters.

- Look current, not trendy—there is never a risk of looking outdated, stuffy, or silly when each detail is considered.

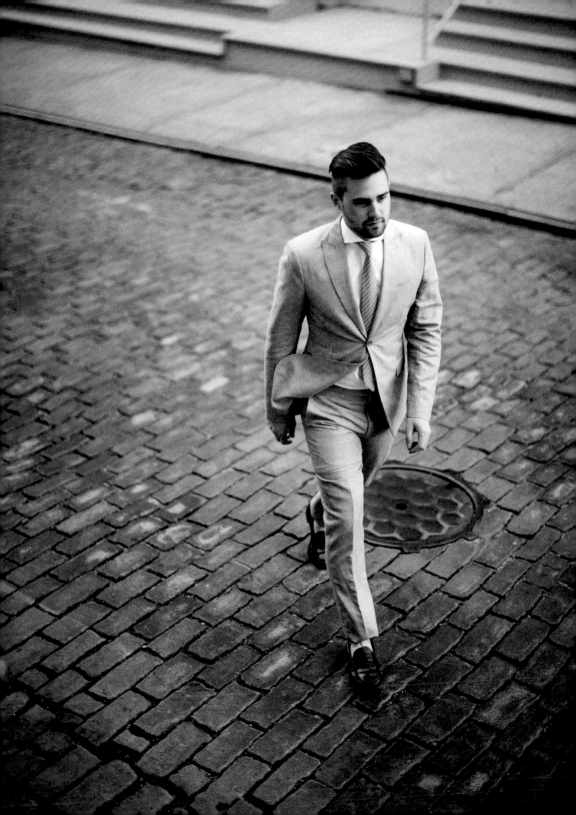

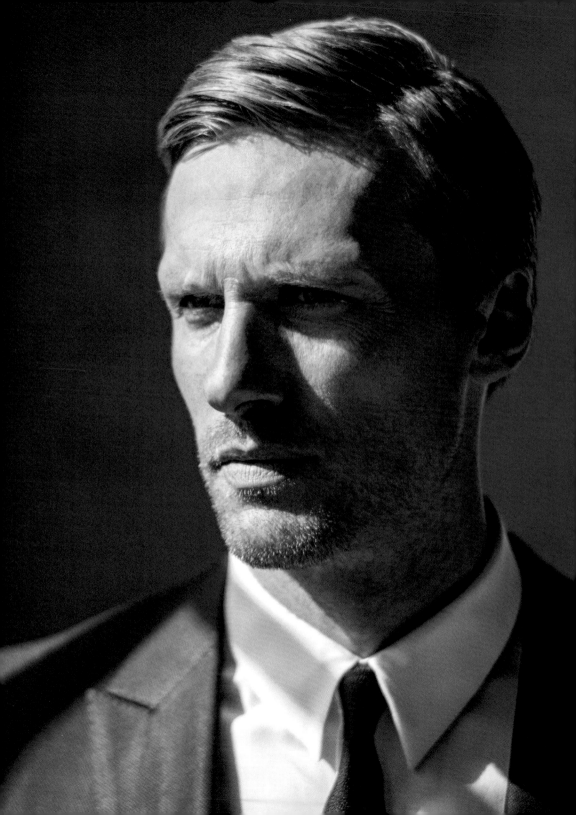

TEDDY SEARS: THE SALGARDO INTERVIEW

F rom the most popular television series to late-night skits, from short films to breakthrough shows, Teddy Sears is one sought-after actor with a wide-ranging appeal. But in his everyday world, he is a gentleman among us and brings a natural ease to his life and style and those around him. We were able to sit down and reconnect after he finished a long shoot and just before a national charity fund-raising trip. He shared his thoughts on finding your voice and look, and how to maintain a well-mannered approach to life.

CHRIS SALGARDO How would you describe your style?

TEDDY SEARS I gravitate towards simple, clean, utilitarian, and always well-made clothing. It's important to have the right silhouette, especially for me since I am tall. There are always interesting trends, but I go for a tried-and-true approach, like the gentlemen of the 1940s and 1950s. You don't need much to achieve a clean, effortless look.

CS Best advice you can give?

TS Finding your own views and voice is one of the great, fun things we can do in life. And I think learning how to dress and build your own style is part of that. So I would say "experiment." Go to thrift stores to see what used to be hot or stylish, and what of it might still work today. I also think it's important to dress for how you want to feel on the inside. Use clothing to express yourself, but also to help you focus how you think, act, and feel.

CS **What inspires you?**

TS It's a funny thing nowadays, living in a social-media environment of such widespread self-comparison. It can mislead. So I focus on the friends and company I keep. These are better sources of influence. Through work I am inspired by great writing and acting, incredible costumes and music. I turn also to the joy and history of my family. My grandfather was a vice admiral, and I just got a hat that I saw him wearing when I was young—and I had hunted for it for years. It was just twelve bucks but was a lost piece of my childhood. The things I get to know and experience personally are my best influences.

CS **What is your view on current in-flight etiquette?**

TS I've witnessed some pretty notable things on flights recently, including just impeccably dressed people. They really stand out among the crowd. You can tell it is important for them, a point of pride. Just when I think people might not care anymore, I will see someone who really wants to look their best. When I travel, it is all about preparing to enjoy it. What's in the bag? What's going to help me wake up freshly after sleeping on a long-haul flight? And your finest pair of shoes will keep you comfortable and happy.

"Surround yourself with people who are honest with you and whom you trust. To succeed in life, you need to hear true advice, even if it is unpleasant and personal sometimes."

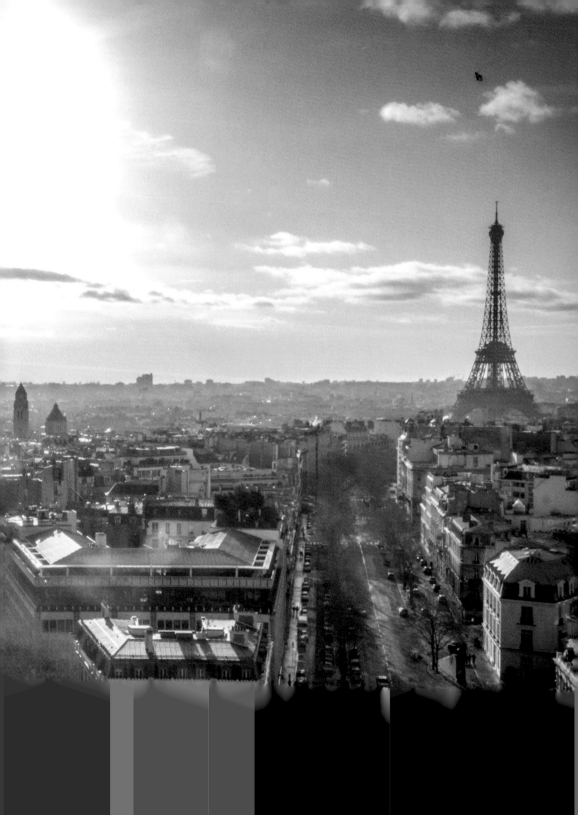

CS **How much does body- and skincare matter to you,
given your career?**

TS Honestly, I don't believe I think about it anymore than other folks. I see my work as my work, and skincare is important for my professional job. But on a daily basis, I take care of my skin diligently. Whether I am currently on-camera or not, I shave to always be ready and sharp. I don't just "pump it up" when the job requires it.

CS **With travel, long days, and the regular stresses of life,
what keeps you focused? Fresh in mind and body, and on
your A game?**

TS My home life grounds me, for sure. I have a calm, supportive, and nurturing family. And my wife makes it all amazing. Like everyone else I try to keep things in balance. No matter how busy, I do my very best to eat and drink the right things, keep a calm mind, and to retain a sense of internal focus. We all have to find and keep our own port in the storm of life. When things get very hectic, I make especially sure not to disappear from the other responsibilities I have. My family. My friends. Exercise and health. The things that really matter should guide you.

CS **iPad or note pad?**

TS Note pad.

CS **Letter or e-mail?**

TS E-mail.

CS Pen or pencil?

TS Pen.

CS What's your most prized possession?

TS When we got married, my wife gave me a beautiful Depression-era Tiffany pocket watch, with the original chain. I know it is just a thing, but I absolutely treasure it because of the occasion.

CS What's your life motto?

TS There is a quote I have on my mirror, above my dresser. It's from Robert Irwin: "It's a constant, continuous, spectacular world we live in, and every day you see things that just knock you out, if you pay attention." I think you have to pay attention and tune in to have a great life. And then I also turn to a line from Chuck Close: "Amateurs look for inspiration; the rest of us just get up and go to work." Hard work counts more than magic. So, I suppose my motto is pay attention and work hard.

CS What are you looking forward to next?

TS I am one of four brothers, and I am looking forward to an upcoming wedding for one of them. And I am actually excited about turning forty soon. As for work, my career is just full of great opportunities right now. My belief is, surely, that the older we get the better we get. So, I can't wait for what's next.

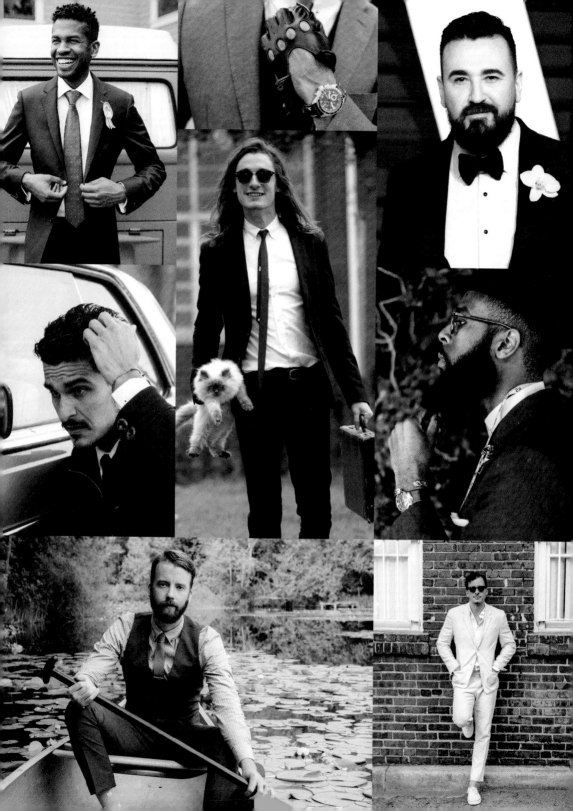

ALL ABOUT THE DETAILS: TOP TIPS FOR THE POLISHED GENTLEMAN

Here's the thing about a truly refined man: He knows exactly when to pay attention and he lives for the details. The crease in his pocket square, his cufflinks, his socks—these small but important touches are never lost on such a fellow. Grooming touches have the same importance.

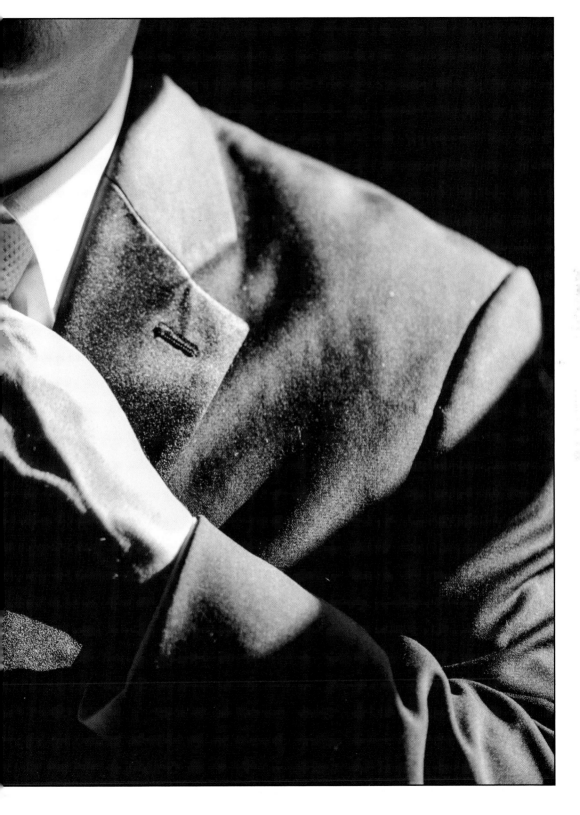

FACE

A good moisturizer will last you from morning to night, but a change in seasons or an overly air-conditioned office climate can quickly derail your regimen. Keep a tube or small jar of moisturizer in your desk drawer. After a full day of meetings, a boost of hydration is just the kick you'll need to go about your evening.

FACIAL HAIR

Give your facial hair the extra love and care it deserves. After showering, apply a dime-size amount of beard oil to your facial hair and work it through with a comb. Allow it to absorb into your skin and hair follicles. This will keep the hair smelling fresh and looking healthy.

SKIN & BODY

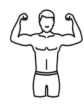

When it comes to caring for your body, give trouble areas such as the elbows, knees, shoulders, and lower legs an extra once-over with moisturizer.

HAIR

Regular cuts and trims are essential to this kind of look, and the only way to ensure that happens is scheduling them in advance, not getting them on an ad hoc basis. Book your appointments approximately three to four weeks out, depending on how quickly your mane grows. A last-minute scramble for a trim can result in a hasty, thoughtless cut, so mark your calendar, set an Outlook reminder, and carry on.

NAILS

Keep your hands and nails presentable with occasional professional attention, and for home maintenance use the appropriate tools. Ditch the metal nail file that can leave your nails jagged and uneven, and opt for a glass nail file instead. Cuticles need moisture as much as the rest of the skin on your hands; rub in some cuticle oil morning and evening if yours are brittle or cracked. Refined detail always happens at the edges.

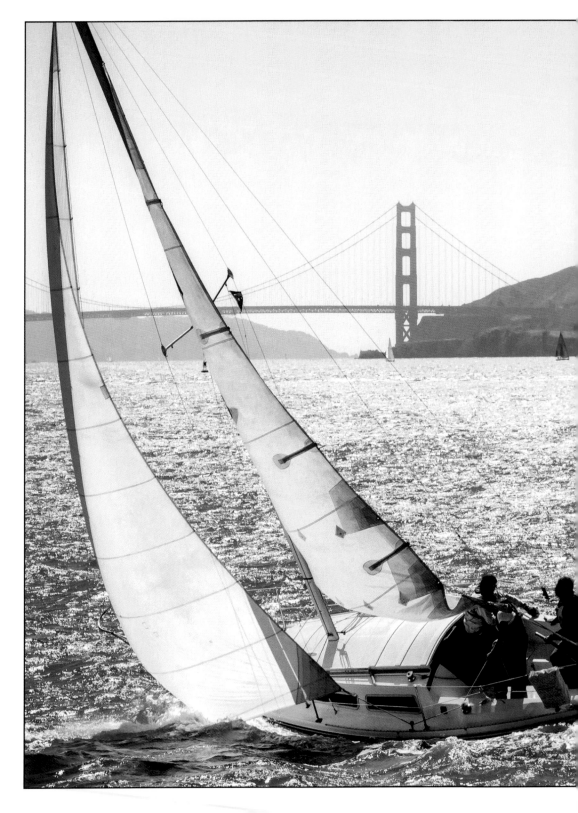

REAL-WORLD REFINEMENT:
A GENTLEMANLY APPROACH TO QUALITY

Keeping things polished and done correctly starts on the inside—with a mind-set, with focus, and with intent. Taking care of yourself is an outward expression of what's going on inside. Delivering the quality you demand in every way depends on a clear sense of beliefs, priorities, and actions that have been considered well in advance, in more reflective moments. The calm and cool moments you take for yourself allow you to give the same to the world.

STAY RESTED

Fifteen- to twenty-minute power naps buff the polish. Not only will you look and feel better, a quick nap refocuses your concentration, restores your Zen, and gets you ready for the next encounter. If a nap isn't possible, lie flat on your back and prop your legs against a wall. The blood rush is good for your heart, mind, and complexion, and is an instant charm refresher.

BUILD FAMILY

Not only your own, but when you travel a lot, you need people who know you and take care of your every need. If you like a hotel or restaurant, book it again. Treat staff well. Remember their names, and they will treat you like family. It makes life on the road a lot more enjoyable.

BE MINDFUL

A smile and friendly hello can go a long way. Don't waste your precious energy on negativity. A positive attitude can be just as beautiful as a perfect appearance; they are all the more powerful when combined.

ORDER VEGETARIAN

Vegetarian in-flight meals may be your best option, as they are often Asian- and Indian-inspired dishes. Better spicing, more vegetables, and fiber are good for your digestion and complexion.

FORGET JET LAG

Step into whatever time of day you encounter when arriving at your destination and go about your business as if you had been there for a week. Don't try to make up for the time lost in flight by napping or going to bed early, it just doesn't work. If you land in the morning, go about the day as if you were at home. Take meetings, work out, hydrate plenty, eat mindfully. Go to bed at night. No naps! Your circadian rhythm will thank you.

CARRY ON

Even if you check your luggage, always have your grooming essentials and a change of clothes in your carry-on bag in case your luggage is lost. Looking good and being sharp is a matter of preparation. Think ahead.

ASK QUESTIONS

Learn from others—cab drivers, waiters, your barber. Everybody has unique life experiences and knowledge that you can benefit from. You will feel more fulfilled and connected to people when you take an interest in their lives, and these social interactions are just as important to feeling good as grooming.

BE PRIVATE

Make a clear distinction between your public and your private life. You give so much all day, a bit of distance is healthy, particularly in the business realm. Some parts of your life should belong to you alone. Let them be your sanctuary.

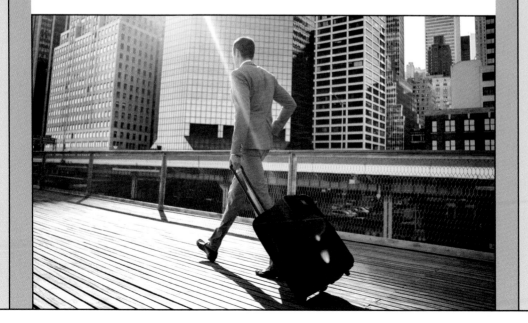

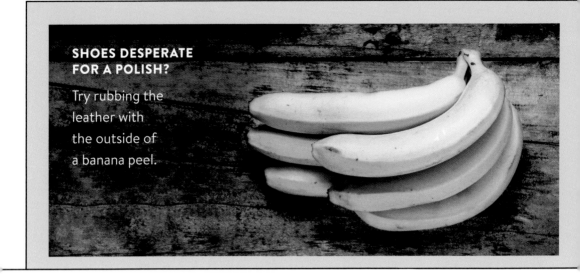

SHOES DESPERATE FOR A POLISH?

Try rubbing the leather with the outside of a banana peel.

STAYING MODERN
WHEN LIFE ISN'T
5 LIFE HACKS

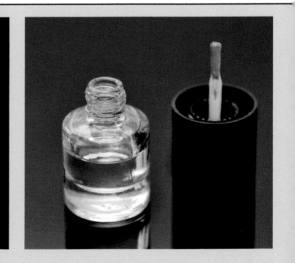

BUTTON COMING LOOSE?

Use clear nail polish to secure the threads before they unravel completely and your button is lost.

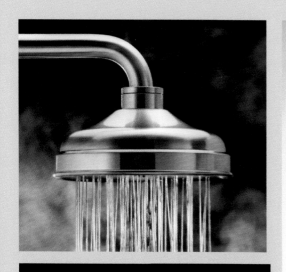

WEAK MAGNETIC CREDIT CARD STRIP?

Apply a layer of cellophane tape over it to smooth out scratches and keep the transaction smooth and efficient.

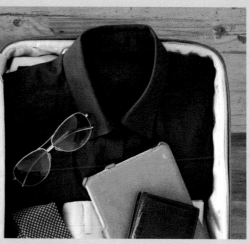

WRINKLES WHEN YOU UNPACK?

Hang your shirt in the bathroom while you shower to steam it before you iron.

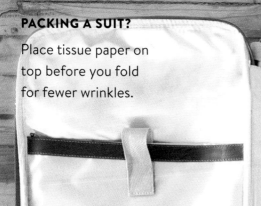

PACKING A SUIT?

Place tissue paper on top before you fold for fewer wrinkles.

GREAT SKIN STARTS . . .

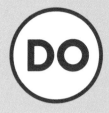

Moisturize. It's nonnegotiable.
Hydration will keep you looking younger.

Use eye cream, and use it liberally. It's your friend.

Use sunscreen.
It's the cheapest and most effective defense against aging.

Use a toner; toners are the rinse cycle for the skin.

Shave with the grain of your hair, not against it.

Exfoliate face and body; it allows all products to work better.

Keep lip balm handy to keep lips hydrated and smooth.

Use a facemask at least twice per month to deep clean the skin.

Use self-tanners to give your skin a healthy and youthful glow.
And read the instructions!

Get rid of ingrown hairs
before they get infected or create skin damage.

AND ENDS WITH THESE BASICS

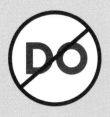

Use rough or abrasive washcloths or loofahs to wash your face.

Use a harsh cleanser or handsoap
that could strip the skin of its natural oils

Use toners with alcohol unless advised,
as they may dry out your skin type

Use a moisturizer that leaves you looking greasy.

Use products not formulated for the eye on the orbital area;
it's too delicate.

Shave with dull blades.

Overexfoliate or strip skin of oils.
You will produce more oil or look very dried out.

Put any makeup products on your face before
you carefully read instructions for proper use.

Overpluck your eyebrows
or pluck the hair above your brows.

Pick at any acne.

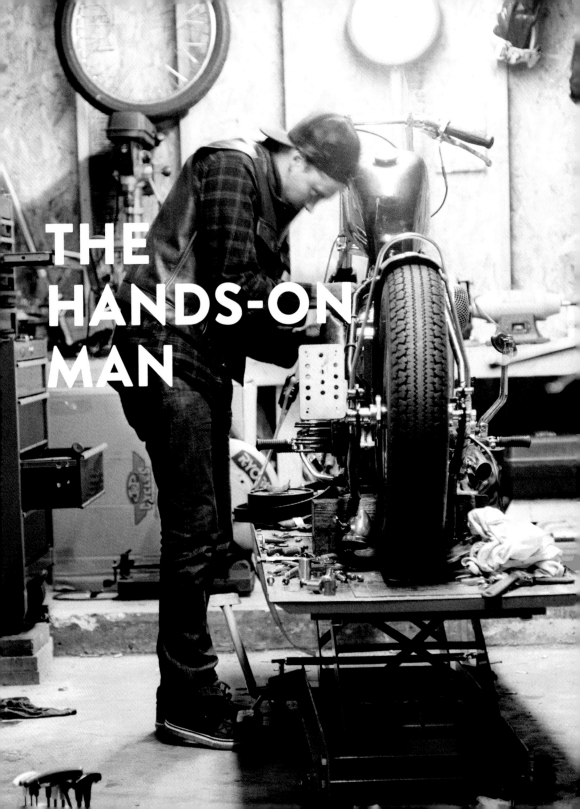

THE
HANDS-ON
MAN

5

HOW-TO'S & HACKS FOR
THE GUY WHO GETS THINGS DONE

Hike, climb, tinker, fix. These are the activities that fuel your fire.

Some guys just have a perpetual drive to modify, improve, motor, and move. It sets them apart from the pack, but that's not why they do it. It's the personal achievement of reaching higher peaks. It's the satisfaction of finding new routes and not taking shortcuts. And then there's the indescribable gratification when guts, gumption, or greasy hands conquer seemingly insurmountable challenges. We all get to be this guy now and then, but for some, it's an avocation. If you're the hands-on man's man among us, chances are we all admire what you're capable of doing, making, and achieving. But that doesn't mean you have the answers when it comes to taking care of yourself.

That impulse to push hard and get the job done eventually takes a toll on your body. Blisters, bruises, and blood . . . calluses, cuts, and mud. You take it all in stride, brushing the dust off your shoulders and keeping your focus on the task at hand. You've bruised your knuckles when the wrench slipped while attempting to break a rusted, baked-on bolt off a beloved bike. You've suffered abrasions from sliding down a trail on your backside. You've inadvertently removed a little skin when working the wood plane. These battle scars are merely proof of what holding strong can achieve.

Maybe you've even performed a little field surgery on your foot with a razor blade, some whiskey doubling as antiseptic and spirit booster— then you slapped on some moleskin and hiked another mile. Rest and healing come at the end of the trip, not along the way.

A teenager heals without much fuss. If skin breaks or blisters, it's no big deal, right? Your body just takes care of things itself. If some part of you doesn't end up wind-burned, sun-scorched, sandblasted, frost-bitten, chapped, or chafed—well, that's a wasted day.

But years of warming your hands next to cylinder heads; waiting until your skin was so cracked and dry it bled; applying sunscreen when it was already far too late; and shrugging off the "avoid skin contact" warning labels on harsh chemicals will leave their marks after a while. The worn leather on your backpack, the perfect patina on the engine case of your cruiser, and the sinuous lines of the table you made from reclaimed barn wood all tell a story of hard work and loving wear, but you don't want your skin to do the same.

We're not talking about losing your character here. We're talking about maintaining yourself with the same care and attention you lavish on the projects you love.

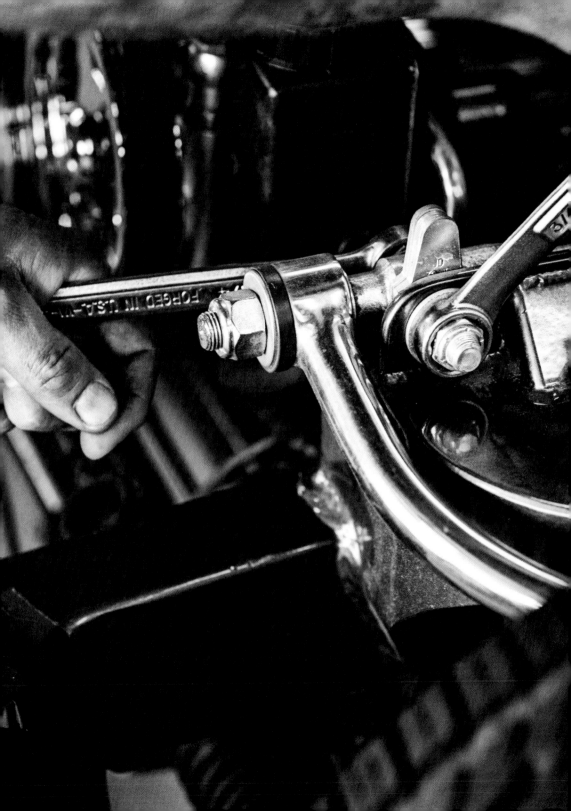

You meticulously sand and stain any wood project before carefully applying even a coat of lacquer. And when you're home from the back-country, you clean your boots and apply mink oil with the care and precision even the most thorough of big-city shoe shiners would admire. It's your stuff, treated your way. That's what makes it valuable. Trea-sured. Real.

So why don't you do the same for yourself? After all, you'll only ever have one body. You can take the same pride in it that you do that clas-sic car parked in the garage. Years from now—when you're a bit more classic yourself—Bondo and sandpaper won't be a viable option.

It's true. Even your MacGyver-like skills can't do much for your appear-ance. You may know less about taking care of your hair, face, body, hands, feet, and nails. I'm here to help. Accepting help may not be in your DNA, but without some guidance your body won't be at its best, allowing you to keep doing more for nearly as long as it should. So just listen for a second.

There's no shame in taking the same amount of pride in your own skin. You're no less of a man for pampering yourself. And nobody will think less of you for conditioning your hair and skin the same way you would the unfinished, reclaimed maple table you lovingly restored to its former glory.

Fortunately, you already know the drill on things worth doing—they should be done right, right? The routine is familiar, even if it feels entirely foreign when *you* are the object of that attention.

Cleaning up is what finishes most good jobs. Use a cleanser to wash your face twice a day—morning and night. Don't use regular bar soap on the rest of your body, which will dry your skin and cause it to over-produce oil. A body wash rich in natural emollients will keep your skin from becoming dry or itchy, and is best for daily use. If you prefer bar soap, be sure to choose one with specific moisturizing oils.

Exfoliating will help get the deeper grime off, in addition to removing dead skin and pollutants from your face and body. It helps keep your pores open and functioning properly to maintain skin's moisture. Go for the deeper clean 2 or 3 times a week but not more; using an exfoliant every day can actually damage your skin.

Making things last means protecting them in the first place—and giving them a little extra loving care if they've been worked especially hard. Think of that old-time catcher's mitt handed down from your grandfather. Your skin needs moisture and protection to stay healthy, so *do* moisturize every day. By supplying what your skin needs each day, you'll ensure it stays healthy and looks its best.

Protect your face before you leave the house. The sun gives life—and breaks it down. But with a touch of preventive maintenance, you can keep solar rays at bay to ensure years of mint condition. There may be nothing more crucially important to your appearance or your health than keeping the sun's blistering effects in check. Winter or summer, sunscreen is a daily requirement. Fortunately, many moisturizers include an SPF ingredient in their formulations, saving you a step. If you don't do anything else to take care of yourself, use a daily moisturizer with sun protection of at least SPF 50. And if you're going to be in the blazing sun for a long time, use a dedicated sunscreen of SPF 50 or more.

When washing your hair, lather up *and* condition. Every time you wash it, you reduce your hair's body and sheen. A great conditioner goes a long way toward helping repair what sun, dry air, and daily shampoo do. Conditioner helps broken protein bonds in your hair to reattach. Your hair will look better if you use it at least once a week. And unless you've been extremely active, there is little need to shampoo every day. Three times per week should be sufficient.

Hands on. Your hands are you most important tools. So give them the same meticulous care you do your socket set, power tools, and lawn equipment. You can't use any other tool effectively if these primary ones aren't in good working order. Clean and moisturize your hands at the end of every day of hard work to minimize calluses. A pumice stone can help remove them. Use a gentle nail brush to remove stains, sap, or grease, if required, rather than an abrasive soap that will damage skin and nails. Apply a richer hand salve during cold, dry winter months to keep skin healthy, protected from cracking, and easier to clean.

KEEP IN MIND

- After a long trail or frustrating project, the haggard look might seem okay to you—but to others . . . not so much.

- Your hands are your most valuable asset—take care of them.

- The sun, the sun, the sun. Love it. Live it. Protect against it.

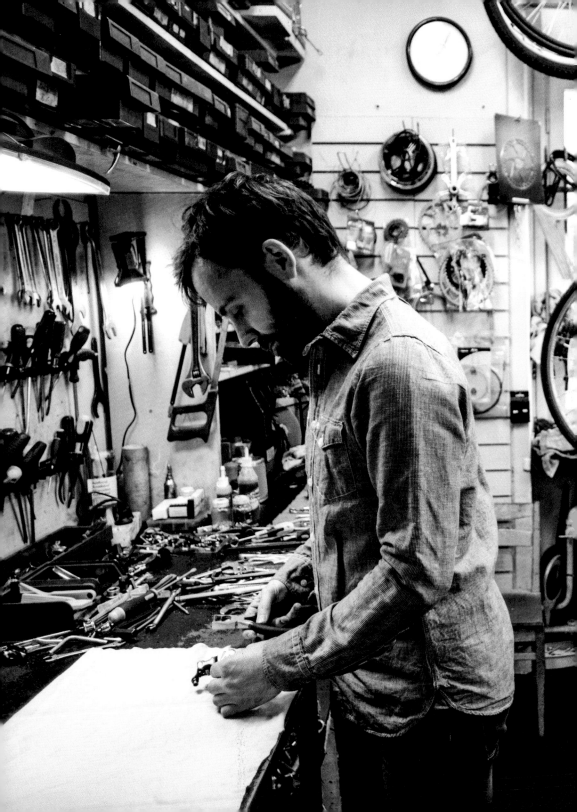

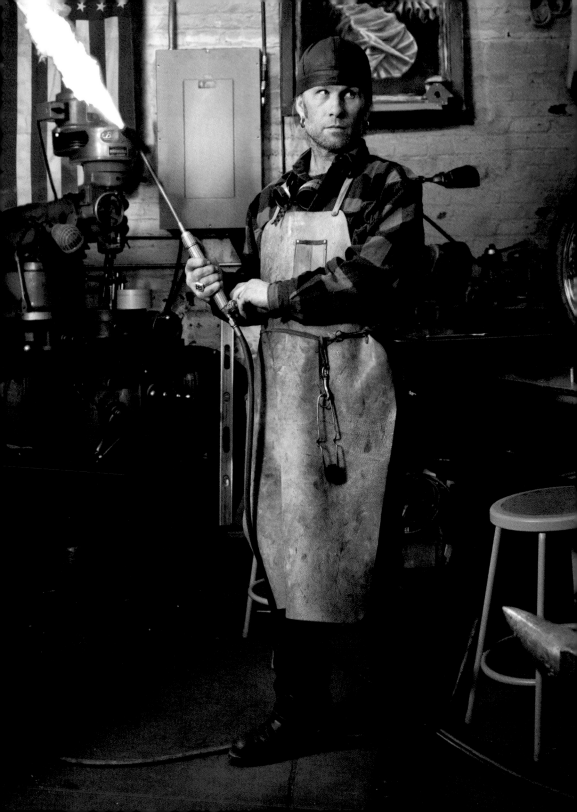

PAUL COX: THE SALGARDO INTERVIEW

Amotorcycle builder, leather craftsman, metalsmith, knife maker, and inventor, Paul Cox knows how to put his hands to work and bring a vision to life in the real world. He has created iconic bikes, and built a legendary workshop, in Paul Cox Industries. Like any true maker, there's very little he can't do or create. We connected to talk about what it means to build, and how to take care of yourself while doing so.

CHRIS SALGARDO **What's the worst thing you've ever done to your body in the pursuit of making the things you want to make, and in your own way?**

PAUL COX Nothing too dramatic . . . lots of burns, deep gashes, and abrasions, but moving from mind to material reality is not a gentle journey. These are physical machines, and I bring them to life one piece at a time. The deadlines are brutal. The all-nighters don't come as easily as they used to. Your hands get knotted, beat up. And double vision sets in.

CS **We both know that our bodies go through a lot with these kinds of hobbies, work, and overall approach to getting life to bend. What are some of the tools of the trade you've learned along the way that have helped you maintain or repair yourself after a long day?**

PC I should do a lot more. I always had really long hair and argan oil was my go-to so that I could keep it a little bit under control. Then, one day I just buzzed off all my hair. I was exhausted, looked in the mirror, and it felt like just one more thing I had to do. So I took the dog clipper and off it went. Simplifying things, streamlining them, became part of my ritual in that instant. And I keep hand salve around the shop. My hands are my livelihood and I can do very little if they aren't healthy. On the rare opportunities that I get a massage, I always have them focus time on working the knots out of my hands first.

CS **How did you learn the basics early on? Who taught you to shave?**

PC That's actually and interesting story for me. My stepfather taught me how to shave. Just gave me a razor and a few pointers. And when my dad found out, he was really upset by it. He really cared and wanted to have been the one to tell me that stuff. For him, it was a skill to be taught, to be passed forward. I got a lot of my creative traits and drive from my dad, but we didn't get to spend a lot of time together. When we did, it was around things we built and enjoyed. I get why he wanted to be the one to teach me.

CS **What's one bit of advice you'd share with younger men to keep them looking and feeling their best without getting distracted from the tasks at hand?**

PC Well, I can tell you that I've come to that place where sometimes I learn more from young people than they may learn from me. Children are still pure. Young people are still discovering. We can see and learn

"Sometimes I learn more from young people than they may learn from me. Children are still pure. Young people are still discovering. We can see and learn what is new or what we missed through them."

what is new or what we missed through them. As for any lessons I have to share, I hope they come through what I make. Before my daughter was born, I made her a knife, and presented it to her as a promise from me. It is inscribed with symbols for *journey, protection, strength,* and *wisdom.*

CS **With that perspective you're talking about having gained, would you change much about how you took care of yourself earlier in life?**

PC Honestly, I would change very little. I've been very fortunate, and even when I might feel tired and beat up, I still feel thirty inside. I'm fifty. Maybe I would tell myself to scale things back, or at least to have more patience and to pace things. I try to do too much at one time. My family is my priority, but I often feel like a lot of years were lost because of my many creative obsessions. There are so many ideas, things to explore, directions to go. I would try to be a bit more organized, I suppose. Concentration and focus are, after all, the entire point of making something. To take time with the details. Whether at home or in the shop, seeing the details is what makes life so beautiful.

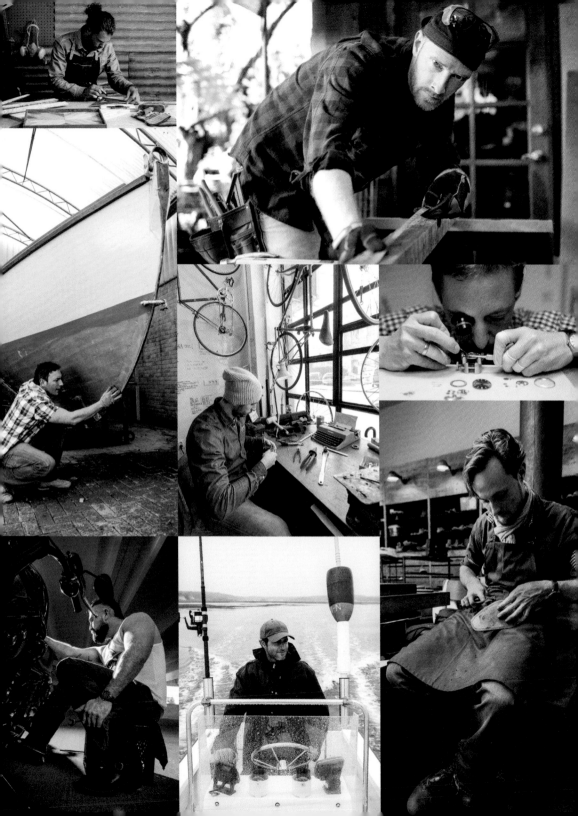

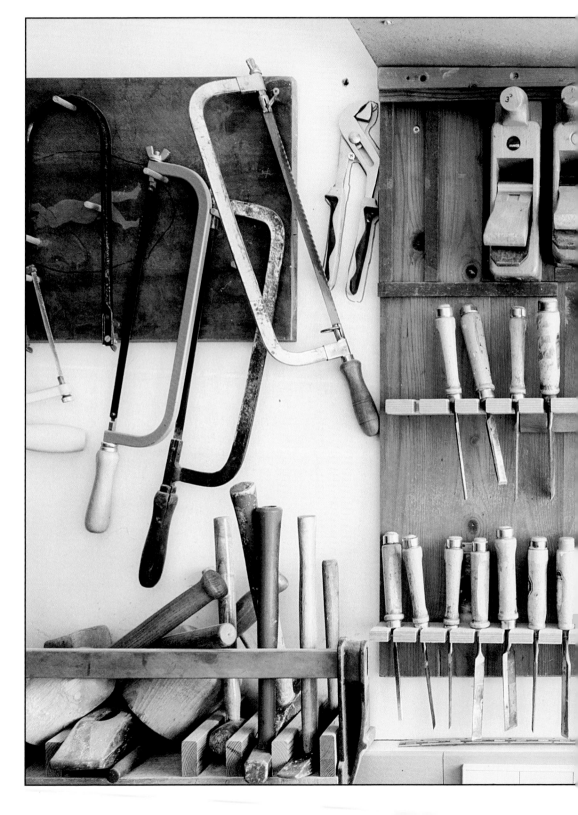

THE FACTS THAT MATTER: ESSENTIAL TIPS

What makes a true man's man? It's an intrinsic understanding of our fundamentals—the ability to get to the root of each issue and fix it in an efficient way without extra fuss. It's about honoring the basics.

FACE

UV rays not only age your skin, but can also put you at serious risk for developing cancer. If you spend less than ten minutes a day in direct sunlight, opt for a moisturizer that contains at least SPF 50. Your skin will stay hydrated, and most important, safe. If you're going to be in the sun for longer than that, you need a dedicated, water-resistant sunscreen with at least SPF 50.

FACIAL HAIR

When it comes to your facial hair, there's nothing wrong with cultivating an au naturel insouciance—but don't *actually* go entirely natural. To avoid stripping natural oils, shampoo your beard a maximum of three times per week, and use a boar-bristle brush to groom it. It will keep your beard looking neat when needed, and will help distribute natural oils across the hair while removing bits of dried food or dead skin cells.

HAIR

Long hours—whether in the heat or the cold—can damage your hair. Consider taking an omega-3 fish oil supplement to protect your hair and scalp from the elements. You'll be amazed at the difference it makes.

SKIN & BODY

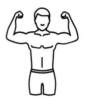

Know the difference between face lotion and body lotion. Body lotion tends to be richer and thicker. Use it liberally after a shower for ultimate hydration. Pay particular attention to the heels and soles of your feet—they go ignored too often and become problem areas later in life. Use a pumice stone in the shower to gently scrub away dead or rough skin.

NAILS

For those who work with their hands, keep fingers and nail beds clean, but don't entirely strip or scrub away callouses. They are there for a reason; they protect your hands against the daily grind. At the same time, there's no excuse for dirt underneath your nails. Hangnails result from unkempt cuticles and are entry points for infection, especially if you work with organic materials. Keep cuticles in shape to avoid fissures and breakage.

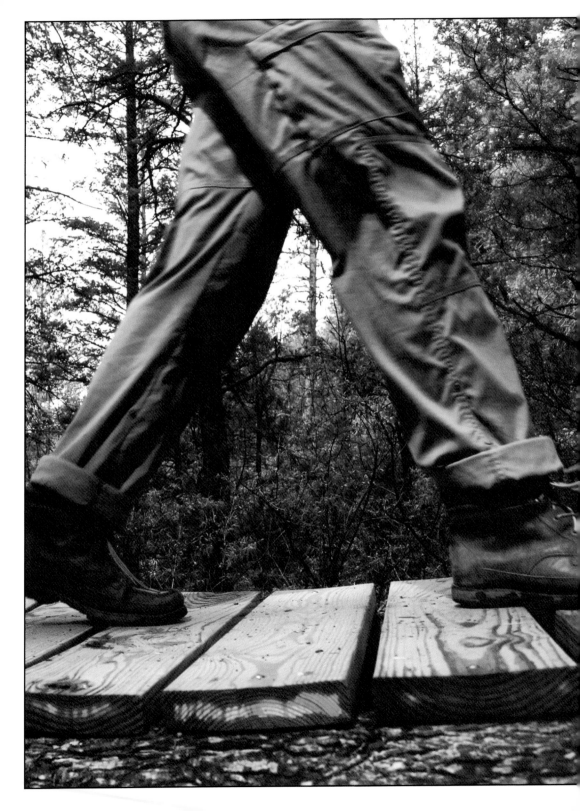

REAL-WORLD DIY: DON'T JUST DO IT YOURSELF. DO IT YOUR WAY.

Taking care of yourself isn't just about how you look. It's also about how you feel, inside and out, as you take life by the horns and make things happen your way. A few important rituals will go a long way toward cultivating your inner quality of life.

LONG DRIVES OR RIDES ALONE

Set aside some time to strike out on your own. Sure, it's fun to go with friends, but there's something more rejuvenating about going solo for a few hours. You don't even need to plan your route. Just go. Go. Always keep water-resistant sunscreen in your backpack or glove box—you don't want anything to stand between you and a spontaneous day in the sun.

DON'T CUT SWITCHBACKS

On the trail of life, it's tempting to go "as the crow flies" when you're getting tired. But that's a shortcut not worth taking on the journey that will be your story. Keep your boots pointed toward the proverbial trail and enjoy life's hike. Sometimes the extra work will not only feel better when you're done, but will have made your body stronger and your mind sharper. And that's what life's really all about, isn't it?

TAKE THINGS APART

This one's a no-brainer. Tinker. Break it down. And put it back together if you can. Just as the joy in life is usually the journey, not the destination, seeing what makes things tick keeps you curious, mentally sharp, and young at heart. Put your hands to work on what others have built. It creates a connection across time.

GET LOST

This might be a tough one, but getting lost from time to time is good for the soul. Lose your bearings. Let yourself go. Finding your way again is more satisfying after meandering about for a bit. But, as you already know, never ask for directions. Figuring things out—including how to get back home—keeps the brain nimble.

APPRECIATE

Appreciate everything in life. Even if something isn't your cup of tea, if others are passionate about it, appreciate it. Your friends and loved ones will thank you. And you will end up reducing your own stress and aging.

PLAY AN INSTRUMENT

Even if you do it poorly, play something. It's fun. It's good for you. Others may appreciate it less, but it's worth it. New things humble us, prove we can still learn, and help us meet new people.

STOP WORRYING

It gets you nowhere. When you're at the end of your life, you won't remember the meetings you were late for. Try to focus on the bigger picture or the specific task at hand. Let the work you care about right now calm your mind. It will show on your face.

SLEEP

Revel in it. Take a day each month to be unrepentantly lazy. You're worth it, and when you are replenished you will have more to give. There is no better protection against aging than consistent, deep sleep.

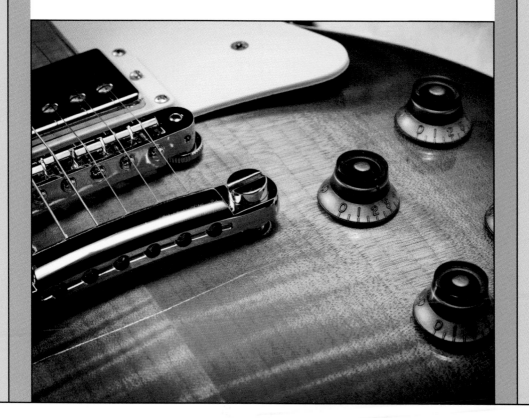

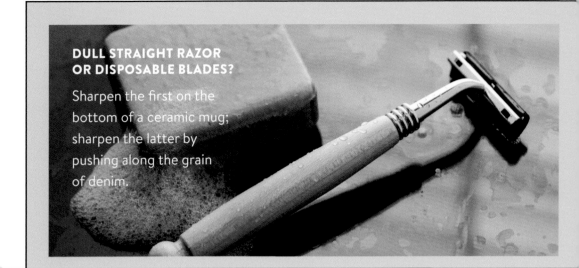

DULL STRAIGHT RAZOR OR DISPOSABLE BLADES?

Sharpen the first on the bottom of a ceramic mug; sharpen the latter by pushing along the grain of denim.

THERE'S ALWAYS A WAY
5 LIFE HACKS

BUGGY CAMPSITE?

Throw sage into the campfire to fend off mosquitoes and stop them feasting on your skin.

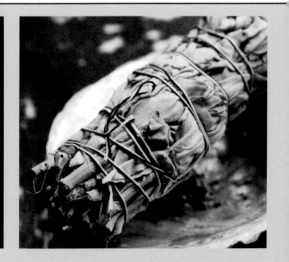

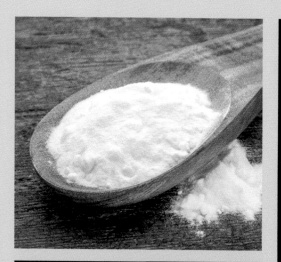

SHORT ON SPACE FOR PACKING?

Roll—don't fold—your clothing; put small product bottles or tubes at the center of the rolls to remove the need of a space-taking Dopp kit.

OUT OF DEODORANT?

Mix cornstarch and baking powder, and rub in vigorously to absorb odor-causing sweat.

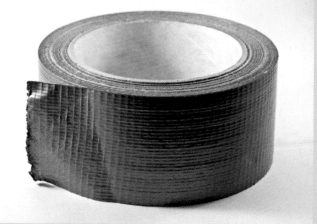

SUFFERING FROM ANY ISSUE AT ALL?

Duct tape. Just duct tape. Set a broken toe. Wax a hairy back. Won't be fun, but it will work.

LOOKING AND FEELING CONFIDENT...

1

Work with what you have. If you are entirely gray, don't dye your hair dark; the maintenance will kill you. The same goes for all-gray facial hair. Fully gray hair and beards generally look better when kept shorter.

2

If you are balding, shaving your head may make you look younger and better styled than trying to hold on to those last few thinning strands. Ask your trusted stylist for a professional opinion before deciding. If you do shave it down, be sure to wear an SPF on that dome every day.

3

Use products that will make your skin look fresh. Key ingredients to look for include: Vitamin C, Vitamin E, and caffeine.

4

Keep your hairstyle clean and modern, but not trendy. Nothing ages a man quicker than trying to look twenty years younger, even if he still runs with the young bucks.

5

Use lip balm and eye cream every day. Visibly dry, chapped lips and crepe-looking skin around the eyes make you look damaged, not intrepid.

AT EVERY AGE

(6)

Use body moisturizer. It will keep your skin youthful and resilient, with much fewer lines.

(7)

Take care of your fingernails and toenails. They can get brittle or discolored as we age. Regular, professional manicures, pedicures, and daily moisturizing will prevent ragged edges and breakage.

(8)

Be judicious with fragrance. You don't want it to make an unintentionally bold statement, or create any reason for distance between yourself and others.

(9)

Get a great dermatologist. Address blemishes, spots, or ingrown hairs professionally to avoid damage. And don't delay getting that new mole or worrisome spot checked out.

(10)

Keep physically fit. You can look athletic at any age. You don't need to bulk up, but keep a tight butt and gut. Diet, squats, sit-ups. And make sure to drink lots of water and get a good night's sleep every day.

THE
EXTREME
DUDE

6

PRACTICAL ADVICE FOR THE MAN WHO PUSHES LIMITS

Setting limits? Not your style.

Slide it, grind it, and spin it . . . jump it, pump it, and win it. You spend hours on end pushing yourself to reach new milestones, riffing off of your friends' best moves, rolling through life the only way you know how: fast.

The difference between winning or losing means having the courage and cojones to get back up after a faceplant to the concrete, racking yourself on the crossbar, twisting your ankle after not clearing that last stair, or getting a mouthful of grit after misjudging a whoop-dee-doo dirt ramp.

Nothing, not busted teeth nor split chins and shins from the tail of a longboard, has given you cause to stop or pull back. You've learned that snow isn't as soft as it looks after over-rotating and failing to stick a landing in the half pipe. You've discovered the importance of good riding leathers after feeling a knobby tire grab skin at full throttle. And you've got the scars to remind you in case you forget.

Let's just say, if the body is a temple, you've been blasphemous. At one point, after several return visits to the emergency room earlier in life, your friends and family may have nicknamed you "Crash." Maybe you've lost track of the broken bones, stitches, contusions, road rashes, and concussions, but your body is still keeping score.

Lance Murdock, *The Simpsons'* resident daredevil, once said "Bones heal, chicks dig scars, and the U.S. of A. has the best doctor-to-daredevil ratio in the world." While there is always truth in humor, the fact is you still need to take care of yourself. Today you wear Rector wrist guards, a helmet, and proper gear to keep your body safe, but it's time to start thinking more about treating the fleshy stuff under those protections with some respect, too.

The inescapable truth is that all of us are aging, and that very fact needs to be reflected in your skincare regimen. You may still revel in skateboards, BMX bikes, dirt bikes, surfboards, and snowboards, but you shouldn't treat your body and skin the way you did when you were in high school.

Before too long, you'll be that "older guy" on the hill going just a little more cautiously than you used to. It's not settling down, it's wising up. It happened to Mat Hoffman, Tony Hawk, Mark "Occy" Occhilupo,

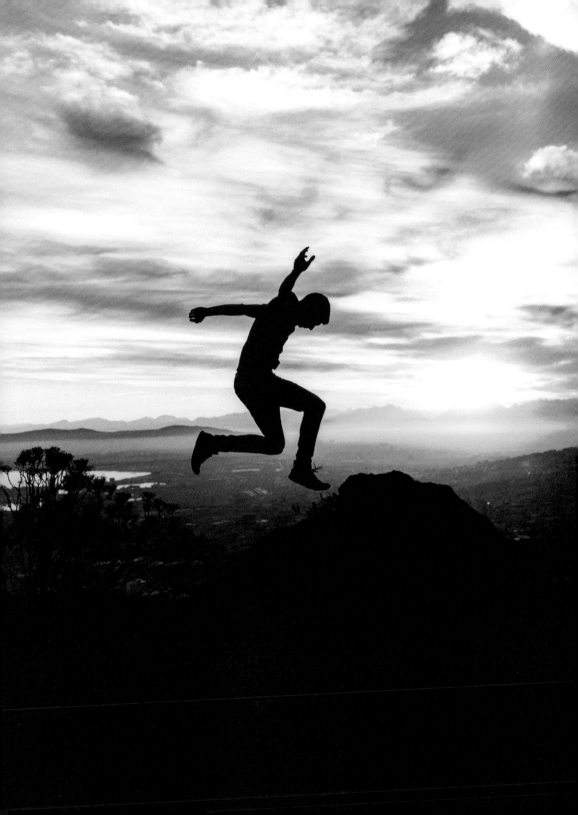

Jake Burton . . . Even Travis Pastrana has toned it down on the bikes, largely retiring his two-wheeled machines to become a demon on the rally track. Whatever changes time may bring, nothing can curtail your passion. There are plenty of double can-cans, backside airs, and 360s left to try.

So keep doing them, and look as good as you can while you're at it, starting with your skin. You've proven what your skin and body can take. It's also important to give them what they need.

Personal grooming and taking the time to care for the body you live in might make you feel a bit less manly—but it shouldn't. And rest assured, the significant other in your life—or the one you're going after—would agree. They can probably overlook—or appreciate—the scars from your ACL surgeries or that time you ruptured your spleen, but looking shaggy, chapped, or just generally unkempt shows a lack of respect for yourself and those you spend your time with. With a little bit of daring and a dose of good advice, you can look as good as that perfect wave, powder-white snow, or freshly built Masonite ramp.

You take care of your gear. The wheels are always well-lubricated and trucks impeccably adjusted. The chain is tightened to factory specs and the suspension height positioned for the task at hand. The surfboard is always waxed and handled with care (outside the water, at least) to avoid speed-stealing dents and dings. Why not treat yourself right, too? You may not see yourself through the lens of your GoPro, but others have to look at you. So do them all—and yourself—a favor. Listen up.

KEEP IN MIND

- Treat your body better. Abrasions are mere flesh wounds, but UV rays last a lifetime.

- Vitamin E helps keep your scars from "tanning" during the summer. Badges of honor don't have to be so noticeable.

- Take care of your hair. Whatever you do with it, make sure it's clean. No matter the style, keep it fresh.

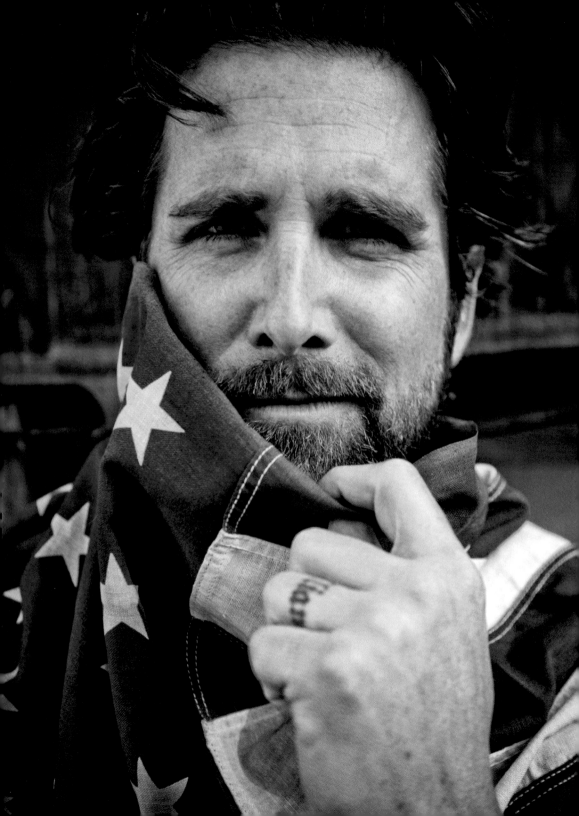

GRANT REYNOLDS:
THE SALGARDO INTERVIEW

A veteran Marine Corps sniper, actor, and host of Discovery Science Channel's *What Could Possibly Go Wrong?*, Grant Reynolds is known for grabbing life by the horns, holding on tight, and blasting through any barriers that dare appear. He pushes himself and all reasonable limits as far as he can. And why not? Moving aggressively forward is the entire point of living, in his view. We chatted about where he got his drive, where he's going next, and how he plans on surviving the journey.

CHRIS SALGARDO **So how did all this energy that is called you come together?**

GRANT REYNOLDS I don't know if it has yet! I think I am legitimately, constantly in motion. I can't stay static too long. It's about growing and going, always. I thrive on a certain type of stimulation. Mind. Body. Soul. Pheromones. Life has to be visceral for me. If it's not, man, I'm moving on.

CS **What's been your worst injury or most physically intense experience with this extreme life-in-motion approach you crave?**

GR Deployments in the Marine Corps, no question. Most people don't grasp how small the Marines really is. Some would say elite. Either way, it's an intense group of pure warriors. You go into it because you have a need and drive to fight for something. I wanted to push it further, so I got involved in the sniper program, plain and simple.

CS **What did it take to recover from it—both physically and mentally?**

GR I was lucky from very early on in life in terms of how I developed physical and mental stamina. Recovery isn't my perspective. I focus on more, further, next. Recover? No. Push past is more like it. I want to win. It feeds me. How far can you shoot? How long can you stay awake? How many miles can you run or bike?

CS **Yet you don't live off in the woods as a survivalist, though I'm sure you could. You clean up well, so who taught you how to shave?**

GR I have a full beard and have had one for more than a decade. Before that, I was one of those Marines who had to shave twice a day to be clean-shaven and ready for formations. Nobody taught me, though. I learned from watching other men shave. You'd watch guys shave sideways, or just their chins. We all figure out some kind of trick or nuance that works for us, right?

CS **Well, we are trying to help guys know the best of that acquired wisdom for sure. Tell me more: What's your earliest memory of trying to take care of your own physical appearance?**

"Honestly, I think the definition of a great friend is **somebody with absolutely no defined purpose in your life whatsoever.** Just somebody you click with, who you fit with. There's no agenda, no objective. Just being."

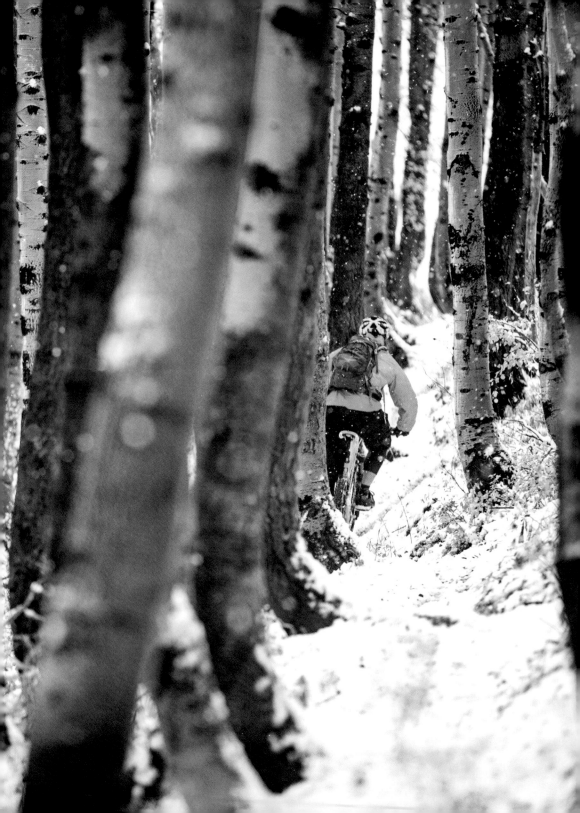

GR Wow. Flashback. It was when my mother got remarried. It was at Little St. Mary's in Fairfax, Virginia. It is the birthplace of Clara Barton, and the American Red Cross, by the way. And my mom wanted my younger brother and me to take part in the wedding. I remember taking one of my new stepfather's razor blades and doing the best I could to clean up.

CS You seem to have learned a good bit along the way. What defines your style, or what do you get complimented on most often now?

GR Good old-fashioned pair of Levi's and a white T-shirt. And I'm lucky to have a nice head of hair.

CS The classics always work. Now, talk to me about your favorite go-fast toys in this warp-speed life of yours.

GR Right now, my favorite toy is my motorcycle, a Ducati Hypermotard 1100S. I like things with wheels and engines. They are the basis of life's best days. It's like a trip to a therapist. I don't buy things to look at or put on my wall. I buy things that have a clear purpose and go very fast.

CS You don't seem to lack any confidence, that's for sure. Anything you aren't wild about, physical features or otherwise?

GR Oh, I'll never live this down. Lips. Honest as I can be. I've got a girlfriend with the most beautiful lips, but I could go for a bit more in that department, I guess.

CS **What attracts you to other people, to friends?**

GR Honestly, I think the definition of a great friend is somebody with absolutely no defined purpose in your life whatsoever. Just somebody you click with, who you fit with. There's no agenda, no objective. Just being. And going as far down the road together as you can. That's how we all evolve, by being on the path together, wherever it leads. And I have to always evolve.

CS **Does anything scare you?**

GR I get asked this a lot lately, given my work. The more I peel that onion, my fears now are my children getting hurt. My biggest fear is my son running out into the street and getting hit. I've got control over my mind and body, but I can't take control of the world.

CS **Speaking of, what advice would you give your son on caring for himself?**

GR It's very simple, and I do say this to him when we negotiate the great battle of teeth brushing. I tell him he only has to brush the ones he wants to keep. Same is true for our bones and skin and hair. I want to make sure he knows he gets one shot at taking care of himself. We all do.

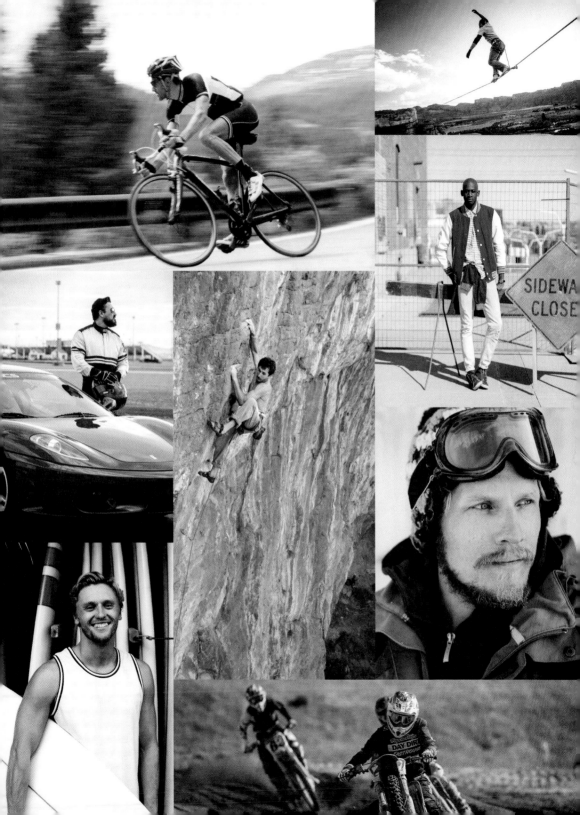

SIDEWA
CLOSE

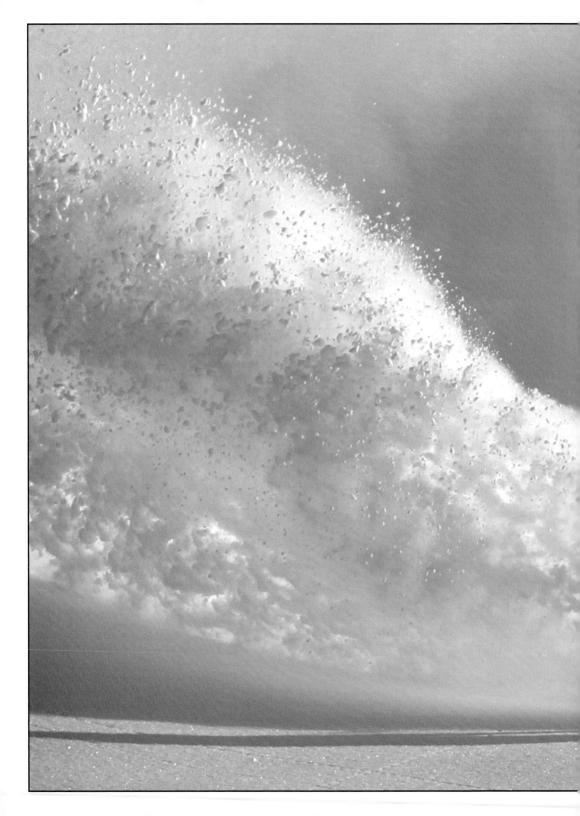

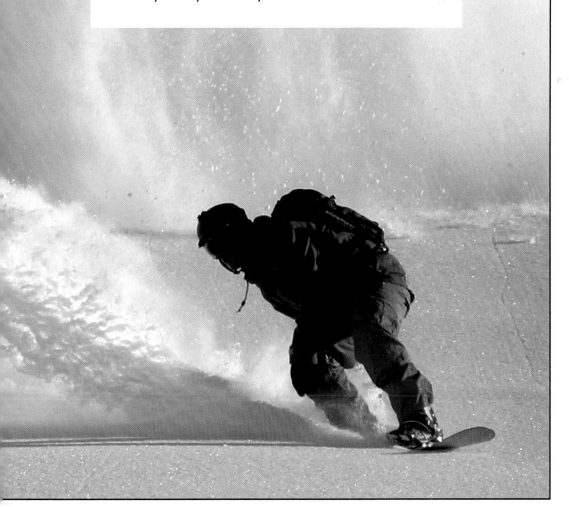

DIALED IN:
BASIC TIPS, NEW TRICKS

For those who lean toward the extreme, it's important to keep skincare and grooming regimens one step ahead, because you, by all evidence, are moving damn fast. From your toes to your fingertips, be prepared for whatever comes your way. And always wear a helmet.

FACE

It's safe to say that your skin is regularly put through the ringer. Sweat, dirt, mud, and whatever else you might blast through will find its way into your pores. Exfoliate your face no more than twice a week to look bright and fresh while not overdrying your skin. Use a gentle cleanser day and night, moisturize afterwards, and protect with a water-resistant, sweat-resistant sunscreen every day. A two-in-one sunscreen and moisturizer will keep this skincare routine streamlined.

FACIAL HAIR

Even if it's only the wilderness you have to impress, set some standards for your facial hair. If you prefer a full beard, be sure to trim your eyebrows, nose, and ear hairs to keep your overall impression sleek and well-kempt. (Note that these will all grow longer and coarser as you get older, so do a good mirror check every few months.) Let all else go wild if you want, but trim around the edges of your beard at least once a month.

HAIR

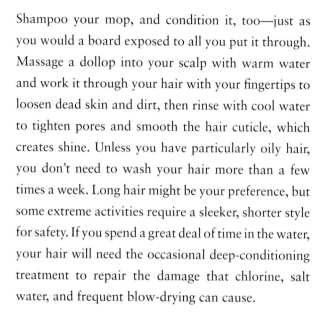

Shampoo your mop, and condition it, too—just as you would a board exposed to all you put it through. Massage a dollop into your scalp with warm water and work it through your hair with your fingertips to loosen dead skin and dirt, then rinse with cool water to tighten pores and smooth the hair cuticle, which creates shine. Unless you have particularly oily hair, you don't need to wash your hair more than a few times a week. Long hair might be your preference, but some extreme activities require a sleeker, shorter style for safety. If you spend a great deal of time in the water, your hair will need the occasional deep-conditioning treatment to repair the damage that chlorine, salt water, and frequent blow-drying can cause.

NAILS

Sure, you may need to keep your hands tough for your next adventure, but there's no excuse for busted nails or cracked heels. Protect and heal nails by using a hand salve on a daily basis. Soak feet in hot water for ten minutes, and then rub your heels and toes with a pumice stone to slough off dry, dead skin. Rub on a rich foot salve or cream, and wear socks over-night to keep the healing warmth and moisture close to the skin.

SKIN & BODY

Become one with the Earth. Place a few drops of blue-green algae extract on your tongue each morning to give yourself a dose of nutrients that will help your skin feel rejuvenated from the inside out, and ready for the what lies ahead. After a rough day, treat scrapes and bruises with aloe vera, and a soak in an Epsom salt bath to relieve your sore muscles.

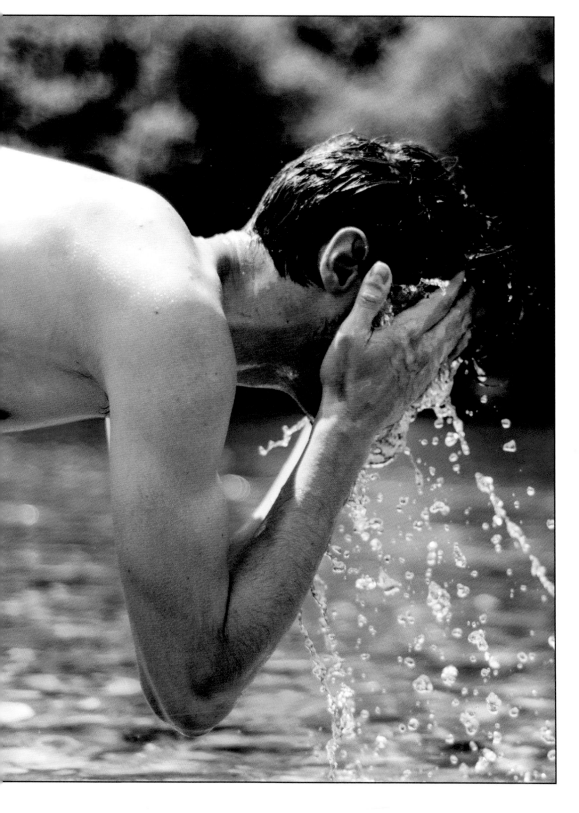

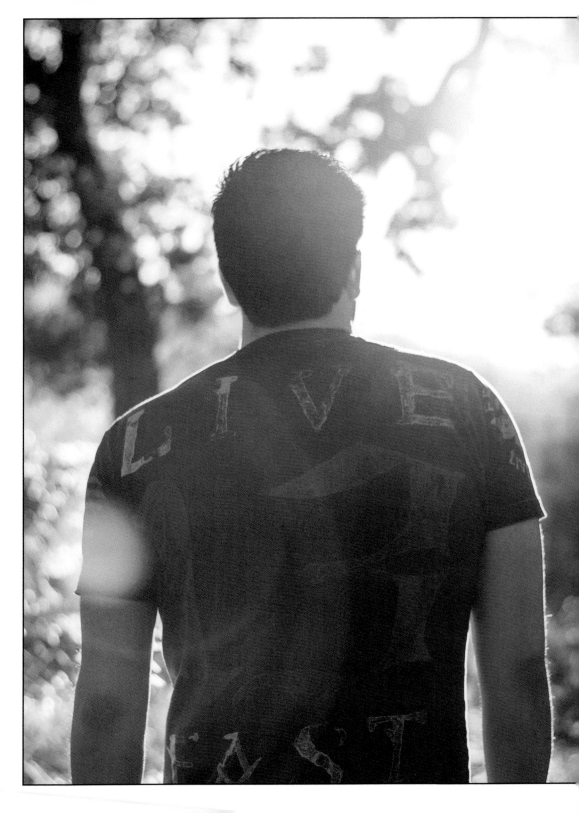

REAL WORLD RAMP-UPS:
HOW TO FIND THE ENERGY TO GO HARD

STAY HYDRATED

And that doesn't mean guzzling down energy drinks, which are packed with sugar. Water gives life. In addition to its benefits for your internal health, it promotes healthy skin, keeping you looking your absolute best.

MEDITATE

Living life on the edge doesn't mean you don't need to refocus and reenergize from time to time. There's no formal training or religious belief required to meditate; just take deep, focused breaths and clear your mind. Relaxation relieves stress, and when you frown less, you reduce wrinkles in the long run.

TRY NEW THINGS

It's easy to fill your free time doing the things you love, but every once in a while, try something new. It will keep you on your toes, and your mind agile. All this translates to greater happiness and a life well lived.

DON'T LET MINOR INJURIES GO

It's tempting to ignore those bruises, cuts, and abrasions. But things that seem like nothing can quickly become something serious. Taking care of your skin means more than just using creams and exfoliators.

TAKE LONG WALKS (PREFERABLY ON THE BEACH)

Besides being good for your physical health, long walks help keep you grounded in the things that really matter in life. They inspire you. They reinvigorate. And as a bonus, walking barefoot in the sand will exfoliate your feet.

GET A PET

Pets make you laugh. Dogs, cats, and other animals can provide unconditional love that's unlike anything else. And a lifetime of smiling and laughter does wonders for both your attitude and appearance.

EAT BETTER

Something so simple can be tough in practice. Skip the double chili cheeseburger and eat something that packs more nutrients than carbs and calories. Not only will it show in your complexion, your heart will thank you, too.

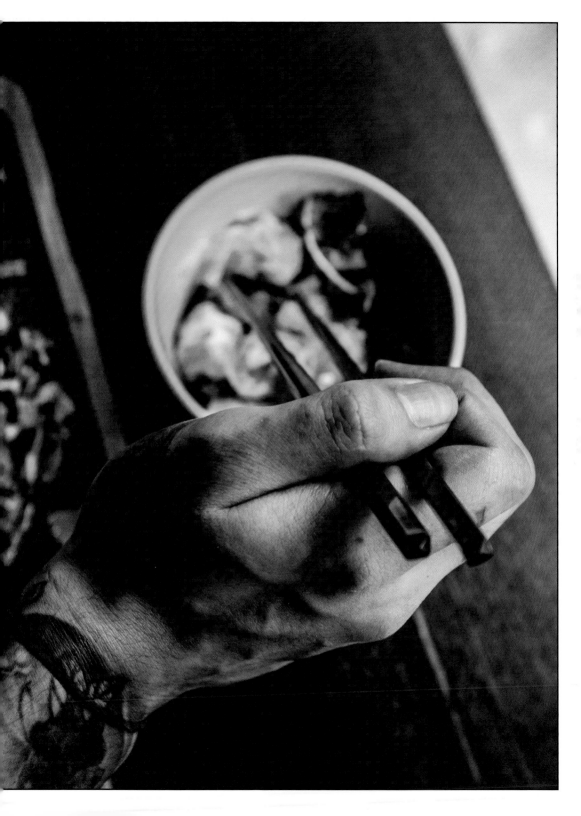

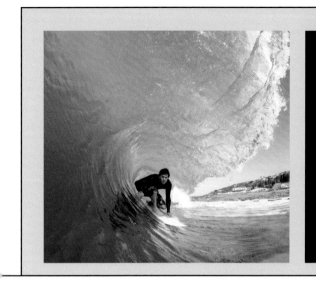

AFTER-SURF WASH?

Keep a clean, gallon-sized jug of fresh water in your car's trunk, and use it to rinse the salt away to prevent skin dehydration.

HIT THE MARK, EVEN IF IT MOVES
5 LIFE HACKS

NEW BOOTS?

Break them in—and pack them out—by wearing them with a thick pair of socks around your home. Even a few hours a week will help save your feet when you finally hit the trail.

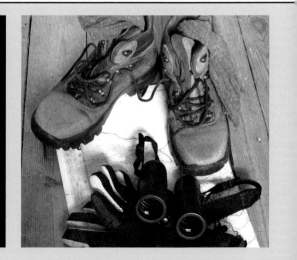

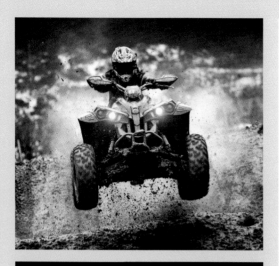

NEED SUNSCREEN OR FACIAL LOTION TO GO?

Fill three-ounce travel size bottles and stash one in each of your jackets or gym bags. You'll never stop feeling pleased with yourself when you wish for some extra sun protection or a drop of moisturizer—and realize you're all set.

MUDDY CLOTHES?

Keep a couple of garbage bags in the bottom of your suitcase or gym bag so they won't come in contact with the rest of your gear. If you're really a mess from head to toe, spread a garbage bag over your car seats to protect them from the muck.

RUN OUT OF SHAVING CREAM?

Try using hair conditioner or body lotion to smooth the shave. Don't use bar soap, as it will dry the skin and increase the likelihood of razor burn or nicks. A steaming hot facecloth held against the skin for three minutes prior to the improvised shave will also make the job easier.

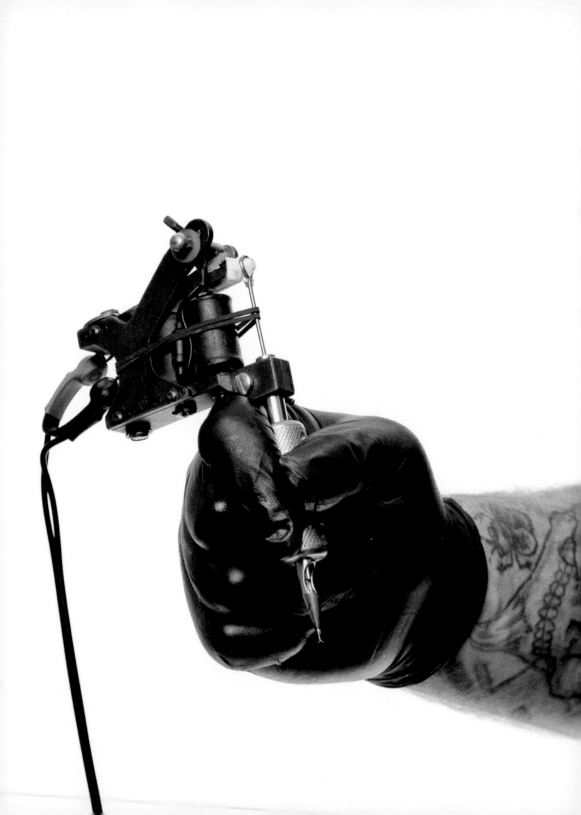

TATTOO AND YOU

Whether you call them ink, body art, or tats, tattoos all require one thing: the insertion of indelible ink into the dermis layer of skin. That's the lower of the two main layers that make up your skin, and it is reached most commonly with a needle. While they've been around for thousands of years and across cultures, tattoos are now more popular than ever—with an estimated one in five adults having at least one. Forty percent of people say a family member has a tattoo.

The best tattoos are the result of care and attention—by both you and your artist. Historically, tattoos often told stories or defined a journey to maturity. And they can still have many meanings, depending on your goal. Do you want a symbol of something that matters to you? To tell a part of your history in a large, complex piece of work? Or simply to feature a decorative element that pleases you? Whatever the answer, intention matters, as the work is permanent. It is important to choose an artist who takes the task as seriously as you do.

If you're getting a tattoo, the following will serve you well:

(1)

CHOOSE AN EXPERIENCED ARTIST

Look at photographs of their work, and see actual examples on other people. Talk to people who have trusted the artist to do their work. Not every artist can execute every look. Some specialize in lettering, others in portraits. Details, clean lines, shading, and strong color are signs of good work. Only use an artist who follows "universal precautions" for cleanliness to ensure health and safety. Ask to see where tools are sterilized.

(2)

SCHEDULE BOTH A CONSULTATION
AND AN APPOINTMENT

Never get a "walk-in" tattoo. Anything permanent on your body should not be done without reflection. And a good tattoo takes plenty of communication and planning. Meet with your artist before the work starts so he or she can sketch and develop ideas for you. Don't be afraid to ask for changes or adjustments. The artwork you approve will be with you a long time. For larger pieces expect several visits.

(3)

CONSIDER LOCATION AND VISIBILITY

Do you want your tattoo to be private, just visible to you and your loved ones? Or do you want to make a statement and share your story all the time to everyone? Full sleeve tattoos can be beautiful, but your workplace might require long shirts to cover it. If you golf, does your club prohibit visible tattoos? Avoid hand, neck, and face tattoos always—unless you've already made it as a rock star.

④
DRINK, EAT, SLEEP

Tattoos do hurt. Don't believe anyone who tells you otherwise. Because they do involve some degree of trauma to your skin, your body needs to be prepared to get one. The day before your tattoo, drink at least two liters of water so your skin is not dehydrated. Never drink alcohol before a tattoo—it thins the blood and dehydrates you. Eat a full meal before your tattoo appointment so you have energy to get through the work and aren't distracted. Sleep a full eight hours the night before, so you can focus and process the pain you will feel.

⑤
SHOWER, PLEASE

While your artist will shave and clean the area to be tattooed, it is a good idea to shower before your tattoo. It will help you relax, and a moisturizing wash will help your skin be ready for the tattoo gun's needle. Plus, it is courteous. Getting a tattoo requires close contact between you and the artist, and neither of you should be distracted by body odor.

⑥
BREATHE DEEPLY

When you hear the tattoo gun growl to life, it will probably be louder than you expect. It's working hard—the needle puncturing your skin between 50 and 3,000 times per minute. It feels to many people like a series of deep cat scratches or beestings. You will bleed some, and the pain can be more intense in certain areas—like near the bend of your elbow or on skin that is often protected, like on your sides. Put on your headphones, turn up the tunes, breathe deeply and steadily, and let the endorphins flow.

(7)
CARE ABOUT AFTERCARE

When your tattoo is complete, your artist will cover it in a thick layer of moisturizing gel, and some type of wrap. It is important to keep this in place as instructed, and then gently wash using an anti-bacterial soap this is fragrance free. Do not scrub a new tattoo with a washcloth or when drying with a towel. Doing so can ruin the work before the skin has healed. Keep the tattooed area heavily moisturized for a full week of healing. Avoid exposing your new tattoo to the sun, and no pool or ocean fun, for at least ten days.

(8)
PROTECT THE ART

The color in your ink—even pure black—will break down over time, and touch-ups may be necessary to keep it looking great. You can slow the process by always applying a moisturizer with SPF 50 over the work.

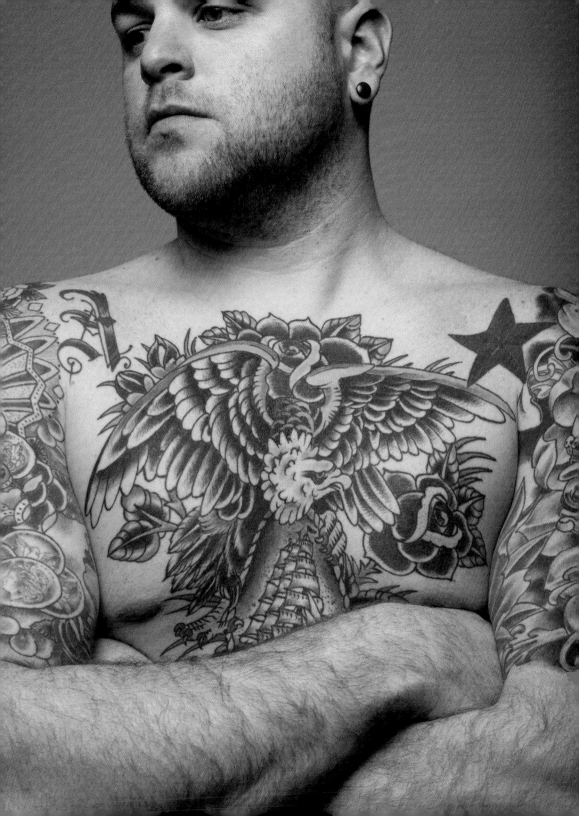

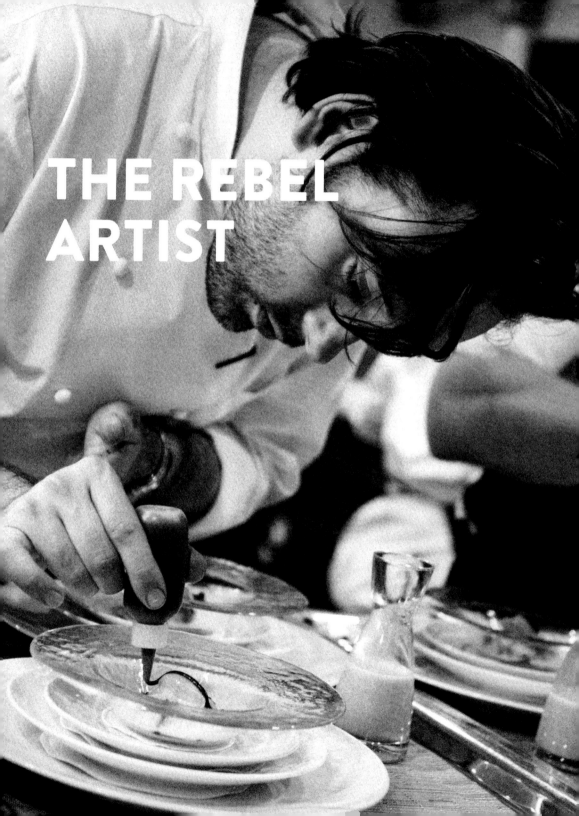

7

A FEW RULES FOR
THRIVING AGAINST THE GRAIN

The drive to question, reinvent, appropriate, innovate, make it up, and make it yours shapes your life. There are too many ideas and too little time to realize them all, but there are two constants—a ceaseless stream of creativity and long nights that melt into workdays and back again.

Your life takes place in crowded venues, hot kitchens, and busy streets, but also in quiet spaces. Almost anything can serve as inspiration, and inspirations are many, given that home is wherever life may take you—across the city, country, or several continents. No matter where you are, your environment is a source of endless stimulation and you are as fascinated by small moments as you are by more outlandish gestures. In some ways, the more surprising and unfamiliar your experiences are, the better.

Chef Paul Liebrandt at work on the line. Photo by Evan Sung.

Image may not be everything to you, but a bold, cultivated air of originality is your calling card. While it is probably not obvious to the outside world, nor should it be, your choices are deliberate and carefully curated.

Fitting in with the mainstream has never been your goal; on the contrary, you prefer to stand out and make a statement. You are unafraid to look, feel, and be different. In fact, that's the whole point.

You love bringing the old and the new together; you cherish the worn aesthetic of your favorite old jacket, whose scuffs and tears are reminders of your artistic evolution, but are equally enthralled by the latest innovations. It's this intersection, this heady blend of time-tested and cutting-edge, that makes your heart skip a beat.

Your work is more than a paycheck—it is a true vocation: personal, passionate, and profound. You give it your all mentally and physically. Your success is based in part on discipline and dedication, but also on respect for creativity and craftsmanship, both your own and that of others. And if not every effort is well received, you have the wisdom to recognize that ups and downs along the way are an important part of the journey.

Your life may be fast and loose, but in other ways it's also deliberate and regimented. It takes both for you to feel at ease. But sometimes the pace of life can be wearing, and can end up etched on your face if you're not careful. That's why carrying a collection of your favorite products is essential. It will let you recharge after too many all-nighters; get ready for that once-in-a-lifetime presentation when the airline lost your luggage; or look your best on that first date.

Fortunately, despite your love of comfort, rituals, and habits, you are open to learning about new ideas. Whether it's a better way to deal with cuts and burns, a new approach to removing paint and grease stains, or a new fitness routine, when you make a new discovery, you break it down and make it your own.

But over the years you have also learned what works and what doesn't. You aren't afraid to say no in any aspect of life. It's been a hard lesson to learn, but now you consider it a personal, earned right. Saying no isn't about being negative or judgmental; it's about knowing what works for you. We've all been there. The lure of a new trend or idea can be seductive, but you and your body are too precious to be treated like a lab rat. Respecting yourself as much as you do others is in your DNA.

You know what makes you feel good and what puts you at ease in an instant: that bespoke piece you bought after your first major success; the small-batch whiskey that's the secret to your perfect Manhattans; the razor set you inherited from your grandfather. It's both about your personal history and trust. Your inner circle is tight knit and only a few gain admission—this applies to the people as much as the advice, brands, and products you invite into your life.

We all know the drill: Time is limited, so anything that takes up yours had better be worth it. You can spend hours obsessing over your latest work to get it just right; debating topics from the latest urban garden trends to that up-and-coming indie band; researching new material or an old technique that may inspire a new project or simply feed your thirst for knowledge, all in search of an authentic experience. You are in awe of things that appear deceptively simple, and know that simplicity represents the ultimate art of life many of us seek to achieve.

You can be intense at times and you have no qualms about it. You have your critics, though you may be the fiercest of them all. You will stand up and voice your opinion, but you are never too proud to accept that others may know more, or to admit when you were wrong. You are able to revise your perspective and consider yourself the richer for it.

Taking good care of yourself is one such instance. You've upped the ante on fitness and diet, but maybe it's time to look more closely, not just at your body of work but also your own body. Maybe it's time for a more holistic look. Maybe it's time to take it up, break it down, and make it yours again, but this time you will make yourself the priority, not your work. It's time to get serious about how you are going to keep looking and feeling great for the next fifty years.

KEEP IN MIND

- Express yourself through both your work and appearance—individuality matters from body to mind.

- Treat the body like a temple, not a laboratory—knowing what works is essential.

- Pursue things that feed body and mind—the art of discovery applies to all aspects in life.

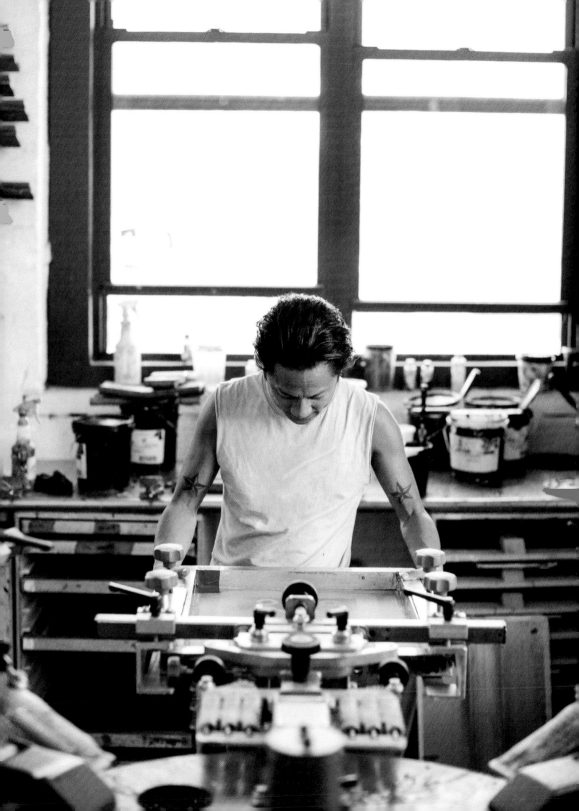

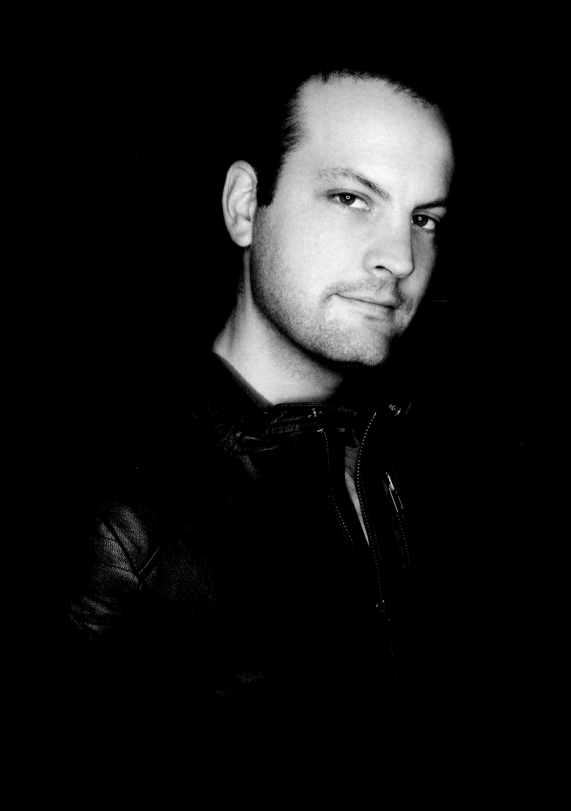

JAYTECH: THE SALGARDO INTERVIEW

A best-selling Australian recording artist since he released his first tracks at just age sixteen, Jaytech (aka James Cayzer) now lives and works in Berlin as an electronic music producer and DJ. He travels constantly on tour to Australia, Europe, Japan, the Middle East, and the United States, and regularly appears at the world's largest music festivals. We had the chance to catch up just as he had put the finishing touches on his next album, three years in the making. We got into how he finds inspiration and makes time for himself while entertaining others across the globe.

CHRIS SALGARDO How did you find your calling? How do you know what you're doing is right?

JAYTECH It all started when I found a flyer on a floor, and I went to an all-ages rave party. I was fourteen at the time, and was totally mesmerized. It set me on my path nearly fifteen years ago, and I've not strayed from it. My parents thought I was going a bit loopy, but it stuck. It was not typical at the time to make music with computers, and I had to convince them my passion was worthwhile. It was the biggest gift, really, to have such clear focus so early on. I never felt lost or on a wandering path.

CS **When do you say "no" to opportunities or ideas that get presented to you?**

JT That's an important question. When your principles are being put on the line you must say no. It is really all an artist has. Their vision and their integrity. I know what's right for my music and what isn't. It's the only way to control your destiny.

CS **What's the best advice you ever received from anyone? Who gave it? And when?**

JT Wow. That's tough. I will say that the most important revelation in a while has been that everything I create is, by its nature, complex. In my music and my life I had too many different things going on. I had to prioritize and focus. I learned the power of paring it down to the most important things, and making those as big as possible. Everything else should surround and support those core things. Whether it is life or work, consolidating and streamlining is one of the best things you can do for yourself.

CS **What advice would you give the younger you?**

JT This is so central to my current album. I would tell my younger self: It's going to be awesome. Just go with it. Stay true to it. And make sure you take time to really see it and feel it and live it.

I would tell my
younger self:
It's going to
be awesome.
Just go with it. Stay
true to it. And make
sure you take time
to really see it and
feel it and live it."

cs **What role does vanity play in your life?**

JT I think being an entertainer you have to accept that your image and face and look are part of your career. There are some who even put this first, building profiles and followings just on looks. For me the music is first, and I always try to portray a positive, forward-looking frame of mind in my work. If it is going to work for me, it is always about looking and being honest. There is a no-bullshit factor to my music, and that has to come through in how I look, too.

cs **What's the best cure for a hangover?**

JT A big bowl of noodle soup. Hands down.

cs **How much did your upbringing influence your style and grooming?**

JT When I was younger, I worked in a supermarket. I remember my dad driving me to work, and my shirt wasn't ironed. He was mortified that I would show up that way. He taught me that how I presented myself could reflect more about me, like my work ethic. I also went to all boys schools, so my style was dictated for me—socks up, a very determined look. So I wasn't as prepared as I could have been when it came time to know what was really my own approach. I've just tried to build my style very naturally, and keep it as simple as possible. I'm not good with accessories or gimmicks. Modest and simple feels right for me.

CS **How do you discover new ideas and things?**

JT All new, creative output stems from experiences you have in life, people that you see, and what you let into your mind. I try to see my local neighborhood in a new way. Take a new path to my studio. Find a new way through the woods on my bike. My tracks get attached to places, experiences, and memories. The work becomes a catalog of what's been lived.

CS **What's your best recent discovery?**

JT My biggest discovery, to be frank, is to slow down. I've always been future-focused, two steps ahead, ready to move on. But that made me gloss over important things. It made me imprecise. In too many ways, I was skipping over important details to get to the destination. The groundwork matters more than I realized. It's really where it all happens.

CS **Take us through a typical day of yours. What are your daily rituals?**

JT I don't know if I have it down to a ritual of specifics. For me, it is how it all adds up. People see all of you at once, not every detail. So I focus on making sure the big things are in place, I guess. I do give particular attention to my facial hair, which grows very quickly. I keep on that every day. And I get my hair cut every two or three weeks, max, and keep the style very simple. I will confess that I keep monobrow at bay with great rigor. Oh, who knows, should I just give up and become one very hairy fellow?

cs **How come your skin looks so good with your irregular schedule, international flights, and many late nights?**

JT Exposure to sunlight is incredibly important to me—especially living in Berlin just now. I try to keep a very strict sleeping schedule to balance out the travel and crazy schedules. In-flight is power-saving mode for me. I listen to podcasts or music. If I am in and out of New York for just a day, for example, I won't change my watch. But if it is more than a two days, I will shift time. Really, it is all about creating order out of chaos, reserving energy, and lots of sleep and water.

cs **What's your ultimate way to relax?**

JT Incredible sushi with great friends, followed by a bit of mischief, if the night goes my way.

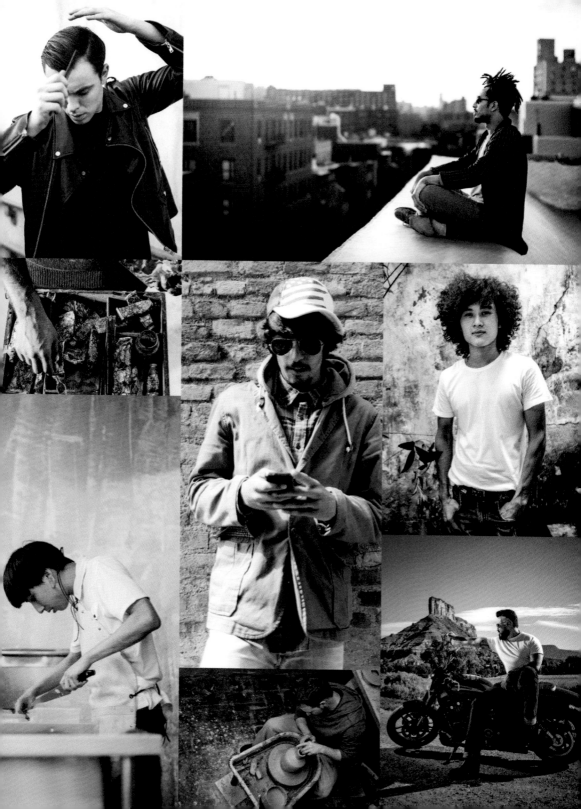

DOING IT YOUR WAY: A FEW INSIDER TRICKS

For true artists, the creative spirit exists in every facet of life. Make an active effort to apply this attitude to your appearance as well. Let your look be a direct reflection of the craft to which you are so devoted.

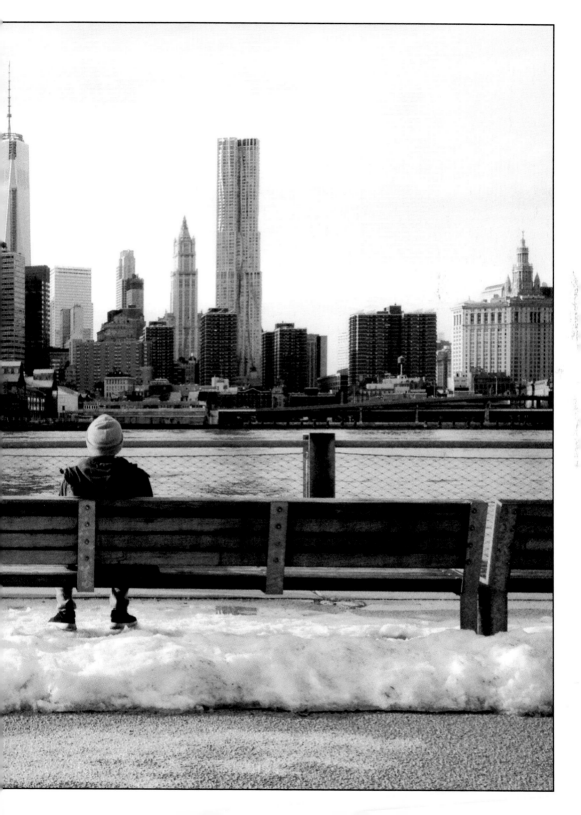

FACE

Pursuing the new can be invigorating but it can also tax your eyes and skin. If you stay up late at the studio or become engrossed in conversation over drinks on a regular basis, pay extra attention to the under-eye area, and use an ice-soaked washcloth, the next day. A microfine polishing scrub can also help brighten skin dulled by smoke in public places or dehydration from travel; just avoid the sensitive eye area.

FACIAL HAIR

There's a time and place for a long, wild beard. Human interaction may be at a minimum during the height of a busy creative or production season, but once it's showtime, a good trim is in order. If you can, make an appointment with your barber. If not, it's time to purchase a pair of sharp, high-quality beard-trimming scissors or professional-grade clippers. Remember always to trim with the growth pattern, considering your desired shape, and smoothly blend the line between your beard and neck. Use a beard brush daily to keep facial hair groomed and neat, especially with longer beards.

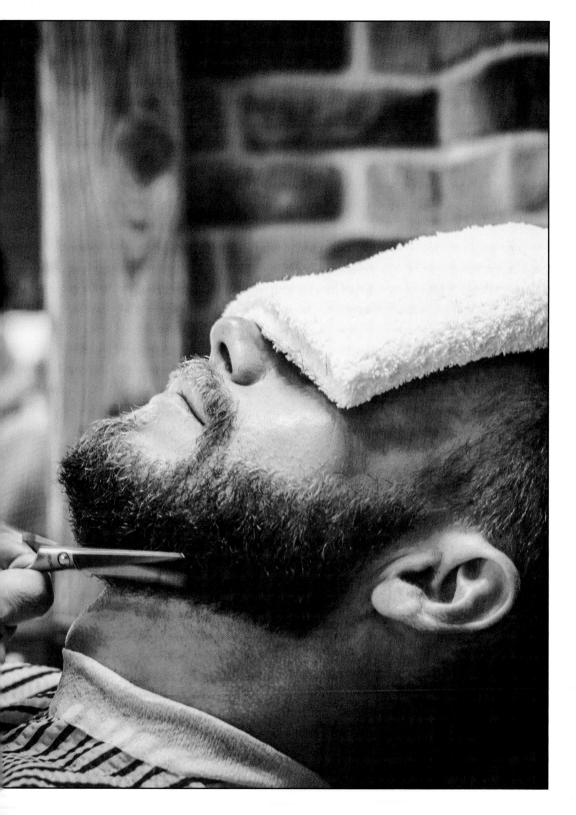

HAIR

Bolder styles, cuts, and techniques can be a good outlet for personal expression, so it's important to find a good stylist that listens to you and that you can trust. Mid-length cuts—as opposed to extremely short or extremely long—will be most versatile for you. If you opt for a more creative style, know you are also committing to adding an extra strong styling cream or paste to keep it in place. Styling with your fingers will create the most relaxed look of all.

NAILS

It's amazing just how much dried paint, clay, or plaster can get stuck under your nails. Leave your work at work, and keep a nailbrush by your sink to scrub away your day's creative residue. Afterward, replenish with a rich hand salve. Alternatively, keep an extra toothbrush for nail care only, and soak fingertips in mild soap and warm water, rather than using harsh chemical agents to remove paint, glue, waxes, or other materials.

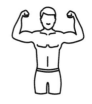

Incandescent, fluorescent, halogen, or LED—it doesn't matter. Indoor lighting just isn't the same as some good old-fashioned sunshine, and long hours in your atelier or working at night can result in a serious Vitamin D deficiency. Consider adding a Vitamin D supplement to your diet to repair your skin and help boost your immune system, and consider applying a vitamin-enriched serum liberally to your face before bed to help restore your skin overnight.

A chiropractor isn't simply for emergencies when you can no longer turn your head. Chiropractic care is part of a holistic approach to health. You throw your body into your work, even if simply by spending hours at the time hunched over a cutting board or at an editing deck. Let your body be on the receiving end of healing work at least once a month. Your lymph, circulatory, and nervous systems all have to work properly to keep you looking and feeling your very best.

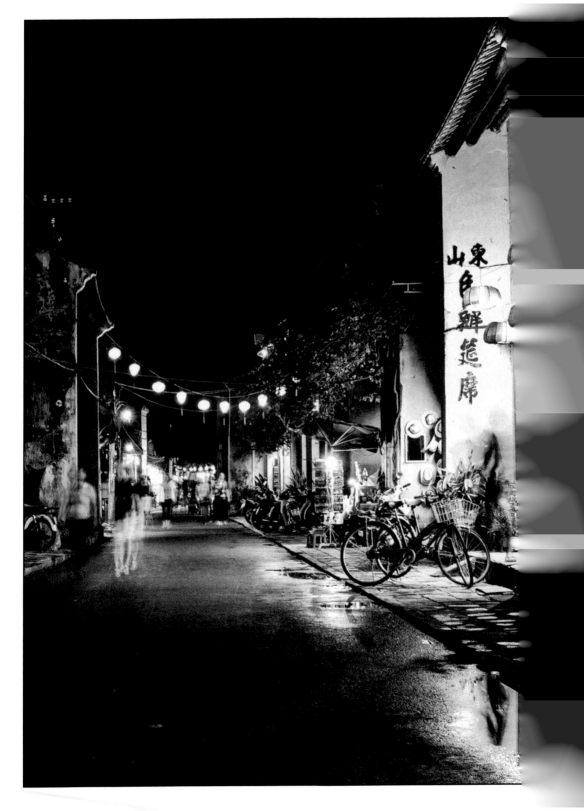

REAL WORLD REMAKE FOR
THE ARTIST REBEL:
LET A LITTLE DISRUPTION INTO
THE EVERYDAY

WALK, DON'T RUN

Walk everywhere you possibly can. Fresh air and mobility are time-tested musts for good circulation and a healthy complexion, and walking allows you to observe along the way. You'll get in some exercise and the discoveries will keep you inspired.

LEARN FROM OTHERS

In a new country, choose a restaurant that is mostly frequented by locals. You will get a greater sense of the people who make this locale unique. It's a great way to absorb the local customs of eye contact, appreciative gestures, or body language, putting you at greater ease during your travels.

DON'T BE A STRANGER

Learn a few words of a foreign language before visiting a country. Even a simple "hello" and "thank you" in the local dialect can open hearts and minds, including your own.

GET CREATIVE

This should be second nature to you. Out of mint? Use the contents of a tea bag. Vegetable bin empty? Treat whatever fruit you have on hand like a vegetable and grill, roast, or sauté it. Ran out of facial cleanser? Turn the shower or bath temperature up a few notches, and let the resulting steam open up your pores.

UNPLUG

Your eyes need a break from glowing screens, so take some time away from technology. The best ideas happen when the brain meanders. Keep thoughts and notes flowing at a slower, more meaningful pace with a pocket notebook and pen. You can type them up or post them later for the world to see.

BE PRESENT

Check in with at least one friend or family member every day, but by the same token, don't be afraid to check out totally every now and then. You'll derive a sense of calm and clarity from being present with yourself through brief meditations, reflections, or prayers.

BE A REGULAR

Find a place to start your day, whether it's the neighborhood park or a local coffee shop. Creating rituals and habits will help you ground yourself, wherever you are in the world. Finding a rhythm, especially when traveling, can help you recover from jet lag more quickly.

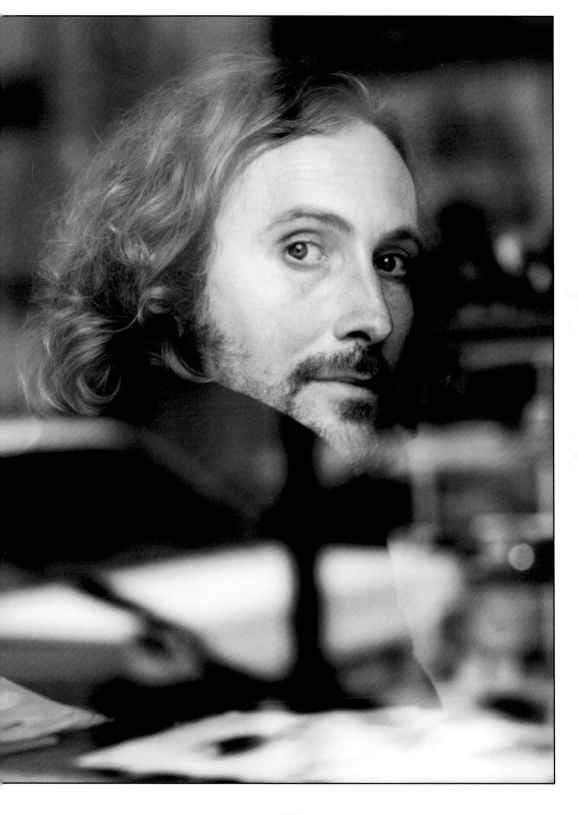

OUT OF HYDRATING MASQUE?

Greek yogurt does a good job, as do a few drops of good olive oil.

REMIXES
5 LIFE HACKS

NEED A SCRUB DOWN?

Mix sugar and lemon juice, and apply in a circular motion with gentle pressure. Avoid the eyes.

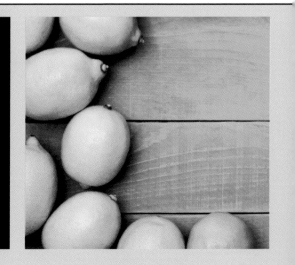

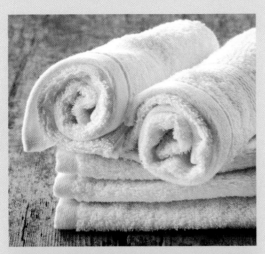

STRESSED AND TIRED, BUT NO TIME FOR SLEEP?

Take ten conscious breaths. Inhale deeper than your natural limit to fully fill the lungs. Exhale longer than you inhale, pushing out stress from the diaphragm upward.

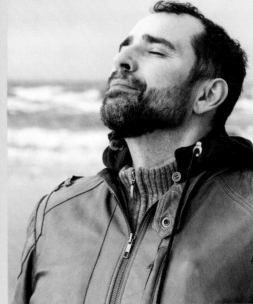

NECK TENSION AND NO TIME FOR A MASSAGE?

Put a steamy towel—soaked in hot tap water or nuked for three minutes in the microwave— around your neck. Roll some fresh herbs inside for bit of aromatherapy. Lavender is calming; peppermint is exhilarating.

UNRULY EYEBROWS?

Hold the wild ones in place with a dab of lip balm until you can properly remove those mother-pluckers.

TRAVEL GROOMING ESSENTIALS

Whether on the road or in the air, whether across the country or around the globe, travel can interrupt your normal skincare and grooming. To stay at the top of your game as you get where you're going, these five simple tips will help.

① DOUBLE HYDRATE

Drink twice as much water as you normally would when flying. Avoid alcohol, as it dehydrates. When driving long distances, remember that dehydration can also occur from exposure to sun and the air-conditioned, closed environment of the car.

② ADJUST TIME

When you cross into a new time zone for more than twenty-four hours, do whatever is normal for local time. Even if your body clock is off, doing so will help you adjust more quickly. For quicker trips, stay on your local time zone to minimize disruption to your natural patterns. A dual time zone watch can help you stay local and track other obligations, too.

③
ALWAYS MOISTURIZE

For flights more than six hours long, apply a clear hydrating serum before takeoff. On long car trips, be aware that sunburns frequently happen through the reflected light of other cars, an open sunroof, or when an arm is rested near a window. Moisturize and protect face and arms with an SPF no less than 50.

④
MANAGE SLEEP

Any form of travel takes extra energy, so sleep when possible. Even a quick nap can help refresh. On long-haul flights, set your watch to your destination time as soon as you board, and operate by it as much as possible. If it is dark when you fly, try to sleep. If it is daylight, try to stay awake. It will help adjust your natural rhythms. Use energizing or calming music as needed to set the mood. Sleep masks and melatonin can be good helpers, too.

⑤
PLAN AHEAD

Before a long-haul flight, give yourself a closer shave so you don't have to worry about shaving as soon as you land. If bearded, travel with your beard brush and use it so you look groomed. Keep a multipurpose product, like a three-in-one cleanser that washes face, body, and hair in your Dopp kit. Pack a small bottle of mouthwash in your briefcase to use when convenient. Use a couple of eye drops to ensure eyes look fresh and rested. Lip balm helps restore lips when dehydrated.

THE RENAISSANCE MAN

8

A THOUGHTFUL APPROACH TO MAINTAINING BODY & SOUL

What makes a man today? You can spend a lot of time thinking about that question. In fact, it might be the only one that really matters. It goes to your sense of responsibility, of integrity, of availability, of strength. The way you answer it at any given moment molds the activities you pursue and the many paths you follow. The answer informs the choices you make.

This might be where your mind inevitably goes on those nights when it keeps you awake, continuing your day's work: *How can I craft a body of work, and a life, that is both rewarding and worthwhile? How can I master the skills I need to make my mark in the way I want to make it? How can I come at things differently in order to create something that outlasts me? How will the world know I was here?*

What is my definition of a life well lived?

Some say it was easier to be a Renaissance Man in the days of Leonardo da Vinci or Benjamin Franklin. When there was less to know, the sum of human knowledge was easier to master in a single lifetime. Things have changed considerably since then. The boundaries of human knowledge have exploded. The sheer amount of information available and its ever-expanding complexity demands the specialist, not the generalist. Do any of us know if we are the right kind of man at this moment in time?

There is always more to master on the way to becoming who you want to be. You will never be able to get to all of it. But to be honest, you wouldn't want to live at any other time. You find it electrifying to be alive *right now*, when you can track the advances in every sphere across the globe and connect with nearly anyone to solve a problem. You have immediate access to more information, computation, and pure power with just your phone in hand than anyone who came before you has ever experienced.

What, then, will you do with it?

You want to think bigger, envision things differently, and avoid the well-worn ruts of how things were done in the past. Some say all the great discoveries are behind us, but the way you see it, the opportunities to define what comes next are nearly infinite.

The individual can have great impact now. *You* can have great impact— and you work daily toward that goal. There are no real barriers except your own ability and mustering the willpower and discipline to sit down and get started. Your determination and ability to focus allow you to explore a subject deeply and enable you to push beyond what others consider possible. You can imagine yourself creating something the world has never seen before or, at the very least, fully appreciating the importance of ideas that others miss.

You take your inspiration from great minds, from the new Renaissance Men who make headlines and history daily. The relentless, restless, curious overachievers and explorers like Richard Branson, Elon Musk, and Steve Jobs define the way we navigate today's world. Does the future belong only to these types of men—the visionaries, the thinkers, the artists, the scientists, and the technologists? Can it also belong to those who can bridge the gaps of our understanding, who can create new insights, who are able to develop new narratives? It belongs to those who want to solve real problems and move us forward, we all hope.

So you consciously nurture an almost irresponsible range of interests and inquiries. You devote considerable time to learning new things simply for the sake of asking the question. *How can architecture and data interact like never before? What will the future of food be like as the climate changes?* You are always interested and curious about everything that is happening in the world today—from space travel to biotech to the latest digital frontiers. The idea of being bored seems downright impossible. New information and depth of knowledge keep your internal fire burning and your mind alive.

When you do decide to mix it up with others, you communicate your vision thoughtfully, with practiced, polished authority—whether in formal settings or simply among your friends. The fact is, for all your solitary pursuit, you love creating an impression. There are moments when *you* can show others something they've never considered before. It's not for ego; it's for the "wow" of seeing the idea catch them like it did you. The man with the idea that wins today is often also the man who can present his idea with the most compelling authority.

You have to make time to nurture yourself as well. What does this mean? The thinking man needs to consider not just his mind, but also his body. If you want to make an impact, you have to look the part. Grooming is an essential function for those who want to create an impression, and how you look affects how others perceive your ideas. That's why having your essential go-tos is critical: a good moisturizer, a razor routine, nail clippers, and lip balm. These simple items allow you to clean up your act, command attention in a room, and move from heady research to real life in one graceful move.

You need to master the tips and tricks that allow you to stand out as boldly as your ideas do, that subtly erase the signs of too many long nights, those tricks that help lend an authority to your presentation. You want to be free to pursue the intellectual life without sacrificing the realities of your body before the final bell rings. As you've learned over the years, in some cases a little knowledge goes a long way.

KEEP IN MIND

- Polished presenters achieve better results. Do your thoughts justice by tending to your appearance.

- Quick touch-ups work wonders. Keep the basics by your side when you're on the run.

- The life of the mind is complemented by consciousness in the present. Observe your rituals regularly.

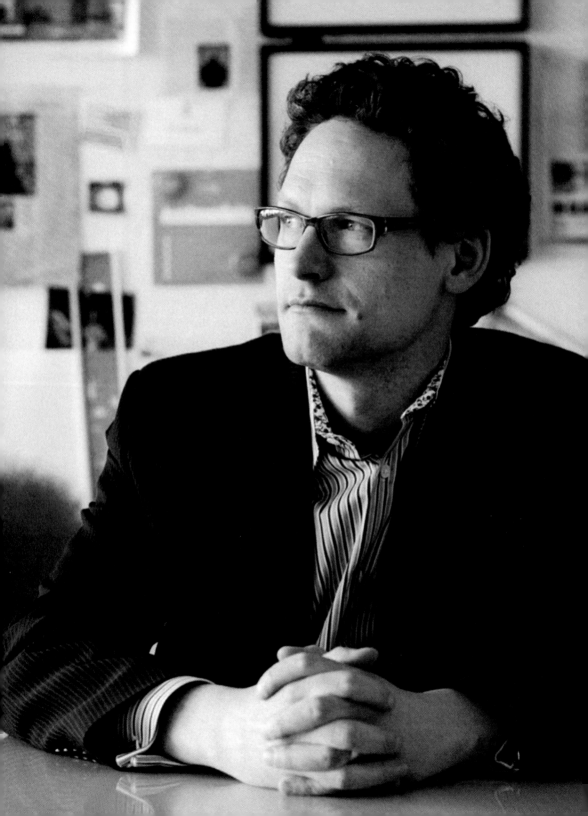

JAKE BARTON: THE SALGARDO INTERVIEW

A rigorous thinker and celebrated designer, Jake Barton is founder and principal of Local Project, a New York City firm focused on experience design and strategy for museums, brands, and public spaces. He focuses on storytelling and technology, and how to use both to emotionally engage modern audiences wherever they may form. He most recently led the media design team for the National September 11 Memorial & Museum. We shared our thoughts and ideas on how to step back from a busy world, see it fully, and figure out what may be coming into focus next.

CHRIS SALGARDO **Why did you start your company?**

JAKE BARTON I'm really interested in engaging audiences through both emotion and technology. I want to give them new ways to interact with art, with cities, and with each other. The communal space is a very powerful space. I've always been obsessed with the ways in which crowds of people, the audience really, could tell the story of the exhibitions better than the curators. Whether it's a World War II exhibit or an exhibition of cars, the expertise in the crowds was always so clear: I wanted to find a way to harness those voices. When technology and the Internet really blew up, I realized that was it, so I quit my job and started Local Projects.

cs **Where do you see yourself going next?**

JB The world is evolving rapidly, but physical space is here to stay. I'm exploring new technologies and new ways to seamlessly change our experience and the emotional resonance of those spaces. Innovation drives much of today's design, but I'm really interested in creating projects that endure. I'm fascinated by how people learn through experience and how we can use technology to help humans be more human.

cs **What's the hardest part about presenting new ideas?**

JB New ideas are always hard to present. When an idea hasn't been seen or experienced before, you have to get the audience to make a leap of faith with you. It's incredibly important to weave the narrative and create a frame—to actually help them see it with you. Sometimes when you don't even entirely see it yourself yet! You're painting a picture of what *could be*. And you have to do it convincingly so that they are willing to come along with you on the journey.

cs **What's the best advice you ever received?**

JB "Try it." That's it in two words. I took that advice and left the theater. I took that advice and started pre-med studies. I took that advice and started designing for museums. Every good thing in my life started with those two words.

"I'm fascinated by how people learn through experience and how we can use technology to **help humans be more human.**"

CS **What would you do differently if you started today?**

JB I can't think of much—if anything, I would be more aggressive about trying things.

CS **Who inspires you?**

JB People inspire me. There is so much poetry inside each of our stories.

CS **How much did your dad or family influence your style?**

JB My father didn't hand out a lot of grooming advice, but I watched him carefully as a young boy, and I've emulated his style. He's a quiet man, but the way he presents is really powerful, and he's been a huge influence on me and the way I work.

CS **How do you discover new ideas and things?**

JB The pace of change is so rapid now, and there are new things all around. I think you have to be still and listen. My instinct is to tell stories. So what I usually do is I wait to see what stories are told to me when I just sit quietly and watch what's happening.

CS **How do you handle critics?**

JB I like the Theodore Roosevelt quote that it is not the critic that counts but the man in the arena. If you're going to live your life according to the words *Try It* you can't let the critical voices get in your way. On the other hand, there is sometimes a lot to be learned from how people perceive your work. I try to block out the noise but listen carefully to the feedback.

CS **What role does preparation play in your life?**

JB It's all about preparation! You simply cannot pull off these kinds of public projects without enormous amounts of preparation and collaboration.

CS **What is your favorite personal care ritual?**

JB I'm a big fan of the occasional massage. I find it rejuvenating, and I use the time to think. I don't get to do it that often, though.

CS **How do you take care of yourself given all the travel?**

JB The travel schedule is the hardest part of owning a company. Trying to be everywhere you need to be without running yourself into the ground. Making sure you look presentable enough to present. I'm a great sleeper on planes, and I am really conscious of what I eat. If I can get sleep and don't succumb to junk food I do a lot better.

CS **What restores you?**

JB My family. My kids are great and I love to watch their curiosity. I learn from them—the way they see and experience life.

cs **What gets your mind going?**

JB Absolutely everything. I don't usually have a problem getting my mind going. It's turning it off that is the hardest part.

cs **So how do you calm down?**

JB I wish I had a good answer for that. I try with the occasional massage. If I have time to work out, that's helpful. But it's a constant struggle to find time for myself quietly.

cs **What's your view on the care of the body so the life of the mind continues?**

JB It's critical, right? I mean, you can't run on fumes. But it's hard to make the time. I do best when I integrate things. Like when I'm in New York I ride my bike to work. I do conference calls standing. If I eat at my desk, it's something healthy. The older we get, the harder it gets. So I'm looking for new ideas—got any?

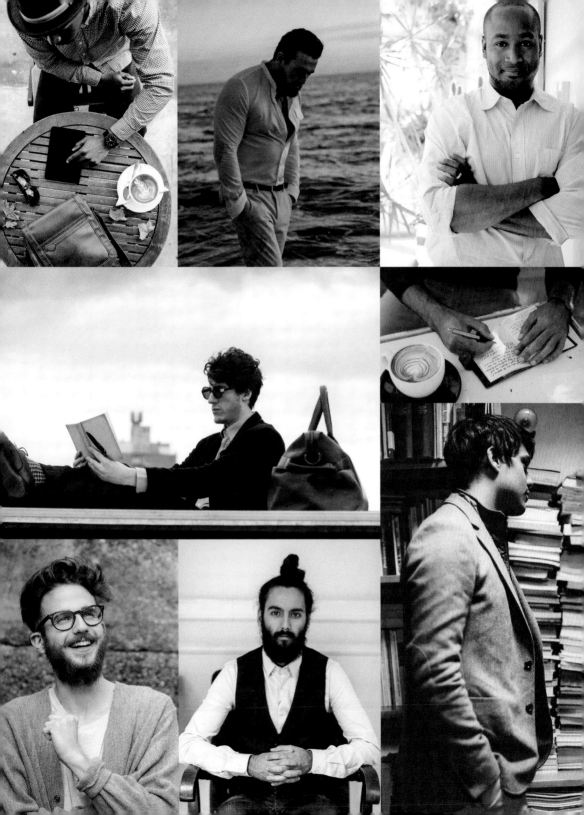

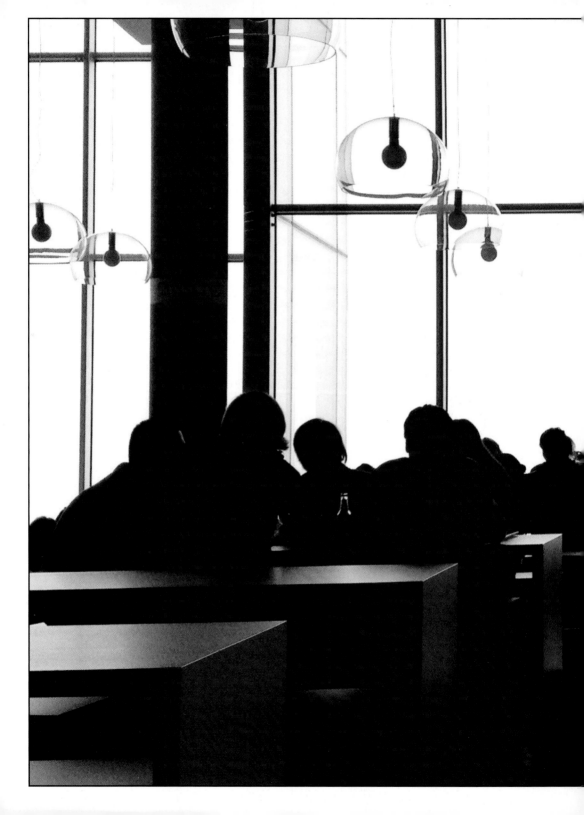

THE BASICS, THOUGHTFULLY APPLIED: ADVICE TO CONSIDER

A strong grooming and skincare regimen is a must for a man of many talents. Don't get so lost in your deep thoughts that you forget to maintain a pragmatic and efficient approach to your overall life and look. Be your very best—inside and out—with these tips and tricks.

FACE

Be resourceful when it comes to your facial skin-care routine. Keep lip balm and moisturizer for face and hands in your travel bag for long flights or long nights. Mists with essential oils are especially good for keeping skin healthy.

HAIR

You never know when life will change its course—or when the price of a last-minute airline ticket to South America will drop. Keep TSA-approved containers (3.4 oz. or less) filled with your go-to hair products in your Dopp kit. Find an excellent hat that feels unique to you for bad hair days.

NAILS

Always keep the right tools on hand. Purchase a small nail kit for your toiletry bag so you'll never be stuck with an uncomfortable hangnail. If you haven't yet broken the habit of biting your nails, at least make sure to file away any rough edges.

FACIAL HAIR

Different cultures take different approaches to facial grooming. One universal "never": the unibrow. Tweeze your brows every three weeks, plucking only from the bottom—and never create a space between your brows wider than the broadest part of your nose. To avoid irritation, apply a small amount of herbal toner or soothing moisturizer where you've tweezed, but don't rub with cotton or other pads, which can irritate the skin and cause ingrown hairs.

SKIN & BODY

Body grooming is a personal preference and can be tricky to navigate, especially when done in the shower. If you choose to shave in the shower, use a transparent shave gel so you can see exactly where you are going with a razor or waterproof trimmer.

Whether you shave or not, be sure to use an after-shower body moisturizer to keep your legs and arms from drying and itching.

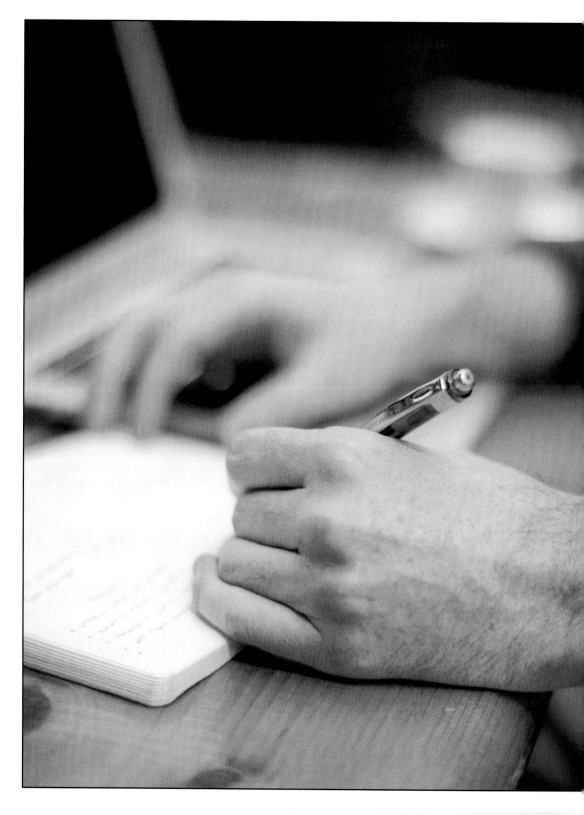

REAL LIFE RENAISSANCE: BALANCING THE INTERNAL AND EXTERNAL

GATHER YOURSELF

Jotting a few words in a notebook each morning helps the mind focus. Take the time to write down your thoughts and ideas as they come to you. The serenity this practice provides—never mind the ideas it collects—will serve you well.

OBSERVE RITUALS

Be mindful about your grooming. Make sure you are completely present during your morning shave or your evening facial cleanse rather than letting your mind wander. Allow yourself to be entirely in the moment. Observe the motions of these small rituals religiously. These self-gifts will provide both physical and mental benefits.

EAT RIGHT

Don't get so lost in your thoughts that you eat mindlessly. It's true, you are what you think, but you are also what you eat. Pay attention to the quality of your fuel. It will propel both your thoughts and your body.

BUILD CONNECTIONS

Assemble a team of professionals who can help you can make your best impression—from clothing to grooming—for important presentations and events.

TAKE A MINUTE

You wouldn't think about taking the podium without having prepared your thoughts, so treat your body the same way. Before you chase down your next assignment give yourself permission to get a massage or a good workout. You'll feel recharged and full of energy.

LOOK UP

Yes, your cell phone connects you to the world's knowledge. But the world isn't only accessed from your phone, tablet, or laptop. Put your device away and observe your surroundings. Make sure your laser focus doesn't separate you from the real world.

LAUGH

There are serious things to accomplish, but there is also life to enjoy. Few things are more attractive than a man with laugh lines. Take time to enjoy this journey you're on. A life well lived includes the pleasure of shared joy.

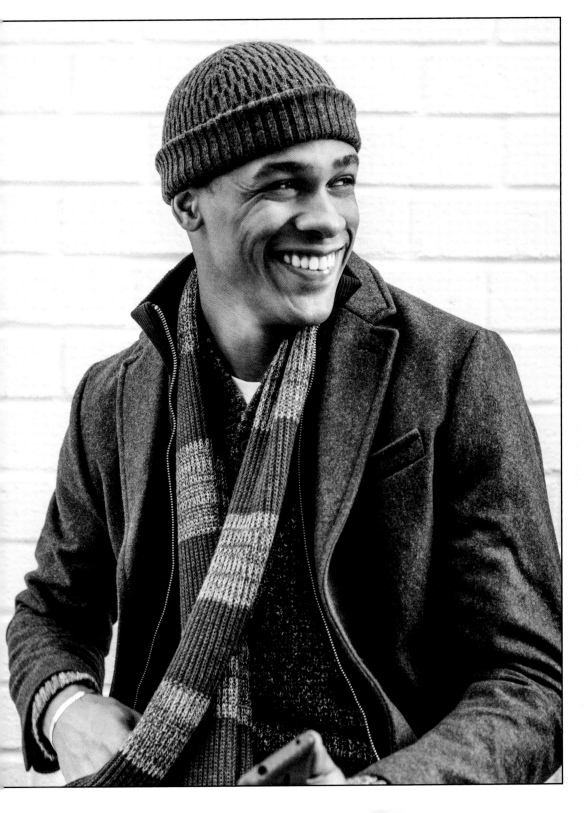

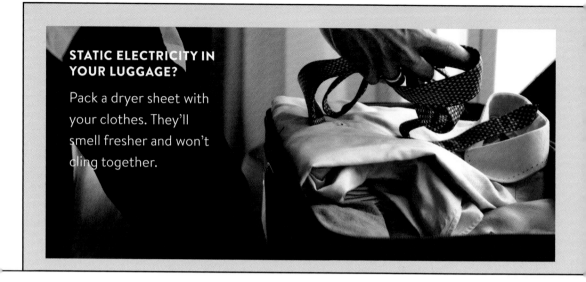

STATIC ELECTRICITY IN YOUR LUGGAGE?

Pack a dryer sheet with your clothes. They'll smell fresher and won't cling together.

FIGURING IT OUT
5 LIFE HACKS

RED, TIRED EYES?

Gently press ice cubes wrapped in a napkin or handkerchief against them for five minutes. Keep lubricating eye drops in your travel bag for a quick hit of moisture, and to keep eyes bright.

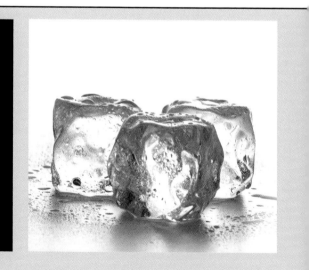

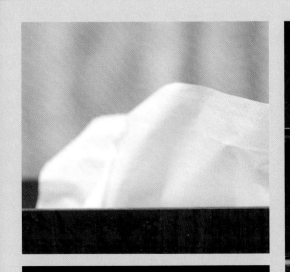

FORGOT YOUR TOOTHBRUSH AND TOOTHPASTE?

Often the concierge at your hotel will be able to send some up. Otherwise, swish some hotel mouthwash for three minutes, then wrap your index finger in a washcloth and rub your teeth vigorously. Rinse and repeat. Buy a tin of mints before your first meeting, and use them throughout the day.

OILY SKIN AND NO TIME TO WASH UP?

Blot your face with tissues: Press for three seconds to remove excess oil from your T-zone. Don't rub, though, as rough fibers can damage and redden skin, and bits of the paper can get caught on your whiskers.

NO TIME TO DO LAUNDRY ON THE ROAD?

Add a breath of freshness by repacking the clothes with a bar or two of hotel soap in between them. Steam out wrinkles by hanging the clothes in the bathroom while you take a hot shower. You will get a day or two of wearable freshness out of them.

WHEN TO GO TO A PRO

Your skin is your largest organ, and good skincare starts at home. But there are times when it is essential to seek the help of professionals. What may start out as something minor—a cut, infection, or mole—can turn into something very serious. If your concerns are cosmetic, there are professionals for that, too. Knowing what to look for and who to turn to matters.

WHEN TO SEE A DERMATOLOGIST

(1) See a dermatologist for anything on your skin that you haven't seen before, or anything that persists—warts, moles, or blemishes that could cause scarring. Don't take an "it will go away" approach. An up-close photo can help track changes.

(2) A medical professional should always evaluate anything red, puffy, sore, or hot—it might be infected. Address immediately anything swollen but without a visible whitehead.

(3) For deep cuts or wounds, err on the side of caution and do so sooner than later. You may need a stitch or two to help it heal properly. And never pick at the area.

(4) Rosacea, eczema, and severe acne are medical, not cosmetic, issues, and require help from your doctor.

(5) If you have a mole that changes shape or color, get to a dermatologist immediately to rule out anything cancerous.

HOW TO APPROACH COSMETIC SURGERY

(1) Remember, less is more on this front. If you do want to explore cosmetic procedures, do so with restraint. A bit over time is best, rather than "a whole new face."

(2) Prioritize anything that may be having a functional impact. Eyelids, for example, sag as a natural part of aging, and can end up affecting vision.

(3) Carefully consider features that erode your self-confidence. A large mole on the face is worth a consultation, but take a moment of reflection before going for the latest trendy procedure.

(4) Approach treatments like fillers with caution. An unexpected result can happen easily.

(5) Look around and ask questions. If you do decide to move forward with a cosmetic procedure, do so based on proven results not marketing claims. Research both the procedure and the practitioner, and then research some more.

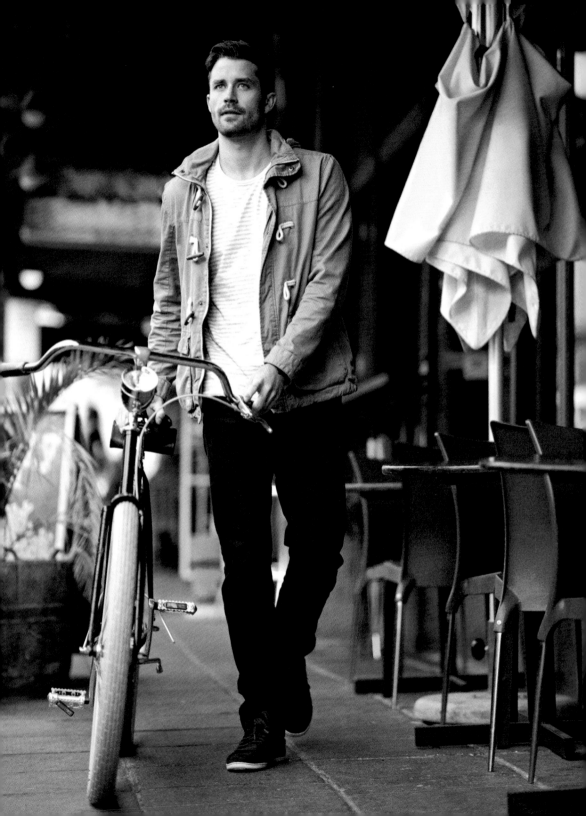

PART III

FOR YOUR QUICK REFERENCE

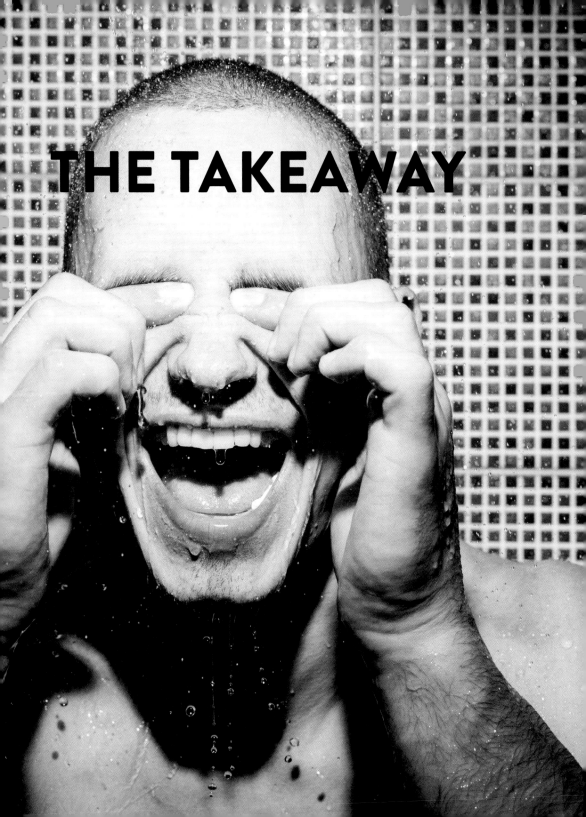

THE TAKEAWAY

9

A ONE-STOP HIT LIST
FOR AN UPDATED YOU

From the questions everyday men ask, to the experiences they have to share, to the professionally proven tips, tactics, and techniques that are sure to work, we have ventured into the real-world of men's skincare and grooming to listen, learn, and report back on what works for modern men, no matter who they are or how they live. Much has been presented throughout the book, and I want it to be easily accessible for quick reference.

Use this section as reminders of the basics, and for a bit of advice when you are on the run. Everything here is explained in more detail throughout the book, too.

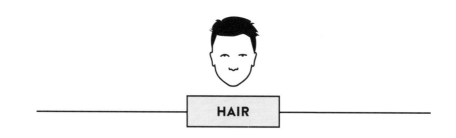

HAIR

- Remember that barbers and stylists can both be helpful. A stylist determines what shape works best for your look and face. A barber can keep things trimmed and tidy in between stylist appointments.

- Not every style works for every person. Make sure to choose a hairstyle that is appropriate for your age, profession, and personality. Longer cuts look most natural and attractive styled smoothly and loosely. Shorter cuts look best when shaped with a stronger holding product.

- Look for hair products with avocado, argan, and coconut oils.

- Shampoo at least three times per week, use conditioner to help repair damaged hair, and consider supplementing your diet with omega-3 fish oil to keep your hair shiny and strong.

- Touch up minor gray on your head or beard yourself if desired, but for anything more than 25% gray, leave the job to a professional. Eyebrows should match the hair on your head, but that is not a DIY job.

- Don't try to disguise thinning hair. It never works. If balding, go with a very short cut, or consider a purposefully shaved head. Confidence is your key to looking your best, regardless. If you are bald, use sunscreen with an SPF of no less than 50 daily.

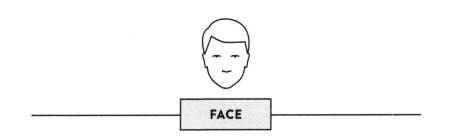

FACE

- Cleanse, moisturize, protect. Every day. SPF 50 or above is essential to avoid sun damage.

- Seek out products with age-fighting ingredients such as copper PCA, calcium PCA, and hyaluronic acid to improve your skin's elasticity. Moisturizers containing squalane will help keep your skin hydrated.

- Moisturizer actually helps control oil production and keeps skin balanced. Use a light moisturizer for day, and a richer moisturizer for skin recovery while you sleep.

- Your eyes and mouth are what most people will remember when they meet you. Keep these looking great at all times. Use lip balm and eye cream every day. And, if needed, whiten teeth with over-the-counter professional-quality products. Always keep breath fresh, too.

- Keep things clean and protected at home. Anything unfamiliar, lasting, or painful means it's time for the dermatologist. Take a "less is more" approach to any potential cosmetic procedures.

- It's perfectly fine to use a bit of self-tanner, bronzer, or concealer to look healthier. But always read the instructions with those products to ensure proper application.

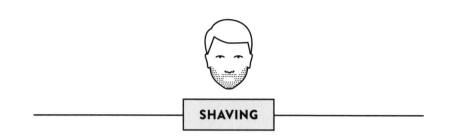

SHAVING

- Always shave with a clean, sharp blade, and always with the growth of the hair.

- Remember to prepare your skin for shaving, either by applying a warm washcloth to your face to soften the beard, or by adding a couple of drops of shaving oil prior to applying shaving cream.

- Choose shave creams over foams. Foams often lack proper moisturizers and can create air pockets that can cause you to nick yourself.

- Electric razors work best for men with sensitive skin or light beards. Those with a thicker beard will do better with a manual razor.

- If you have no important meetings or weekend plans, give your skin a rest. Shaving can be tough on it.

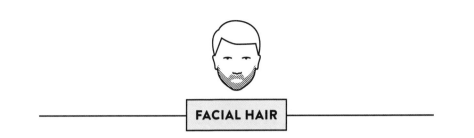

FACIAL HAIR

- Beard shape matters—it can add length to a rounder face or fullness to a narrower face. Think through your beard style, just like you do a hair style.

- Make sure to have a safety razor, beard trimmer, and a sharp pair of beard scissors to maintain your look.

- Use a trimmer to buzz from your Adam's apple to about two inches below your jawline, for a smooth transition into your beard. Use a razor to create a clean line between your beard and your cheek. Scissors are best for cleaning up stray hairs and near the lip line.

- Include beard oil in your care ritual to keep it looking smooth. Choose products with argan oil. Consider a hint of spearmint or eucalyptus as well for a refreshing note.

- Exfoliate any shaved areas regularly to control ingrown hairs. Doing so helps keep pores and follicles from getting clogged and irritated.

- Trim nose and ear hairs regularly, using a battery-powered trimmer rather than scissors. Never pluck ear or nose hair, as it can lead to infection.

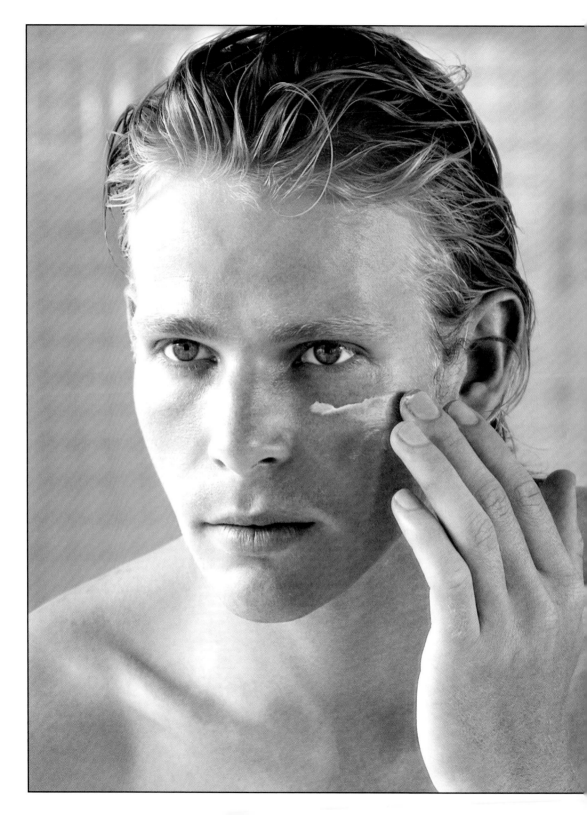

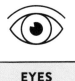

EYES

- Remember that the skin around your eyes is thinner than the skin on the rest of your face, and contains one-third fewer oils. Commit to eye cream as an essential daily step and use products specifically made for the eye area.

- Look for products containing Vitamin C. Using them will help brighten the skin around your eyes over time.

- Travel with eyedrops to get the red out after a long flight. You'll look fresh and rested.

- Place an ice-cold washcloth against your eyes to help reduce puffiness and circles. Seek eye products with caffeine as an ingredient, since it can also help reduce puffiness.

- Keep eyebrows in check. If you pluck, do so between the brows and under them, but never over them, so as to keep their natural shape. Use an eyebrow trimmer with a guard if things get especially wild. A small brush can also help keep them looking neat.

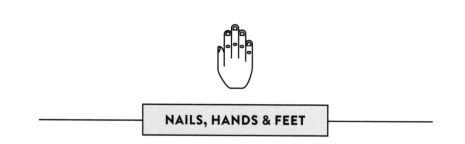

NAILS, HANDS & FEET

- Hands and feet need moisturizing, just like the rest of your skin. Use products made specifically for the tougher skin on these areas at least once a week.

- Always keep hands clean and nails trimmed. Choose a glass file over other options. And get a manicure every two months to keep cuticles trimmed and healthy. A buffed finish, not clear polish, looks best.

- Use a scrub brush or pumice stone to keep rough foot skin in check. Get a pedicure every two months.

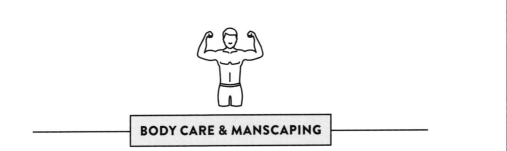

BODY CARE & MANSCAPING

- Keep your skin hydrated, healthy, and in balance with an after-shower body moisturizer or oil.

- Use body washes rather than bar soap to ensure gentle cleansing and proper moisturizing.

- No matter the season, sunscreen is a daily requirement, on arms, legs, and scalp as well as the face. Choose SPF 50 or higher.

- Consider taking a Vitamin D supplement to help keep skin healthy.

- If you manscape, do so slowly and in the growth direction of the hair. Never shave arms or legs, as doing so doesn't look natural.

- If you choose to wax body hair, trim it first. It will hurt less. Only use a trusted professional for this job.

- To control excessive body odor, bathe more often, limit pungent food intake, and consider clinical antiperspirants.

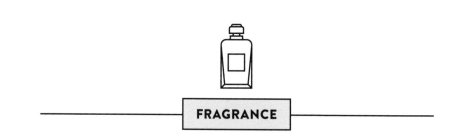

FRAGRANCE

- A signature scent can be a great part of your style. Just make sure it is not overwhelming and does not combine unpleasantly with scents from other products.

- Don't "crush" fragrance notes by rubbing them in. Lightly spray scent onto the sides of your neck or wrists.

- Choose lighter scents for summer and more complex ones for winter.

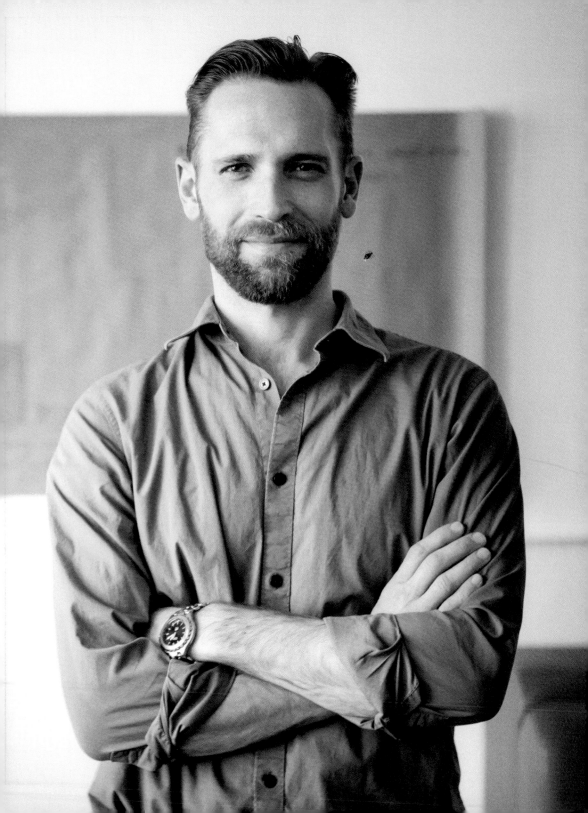

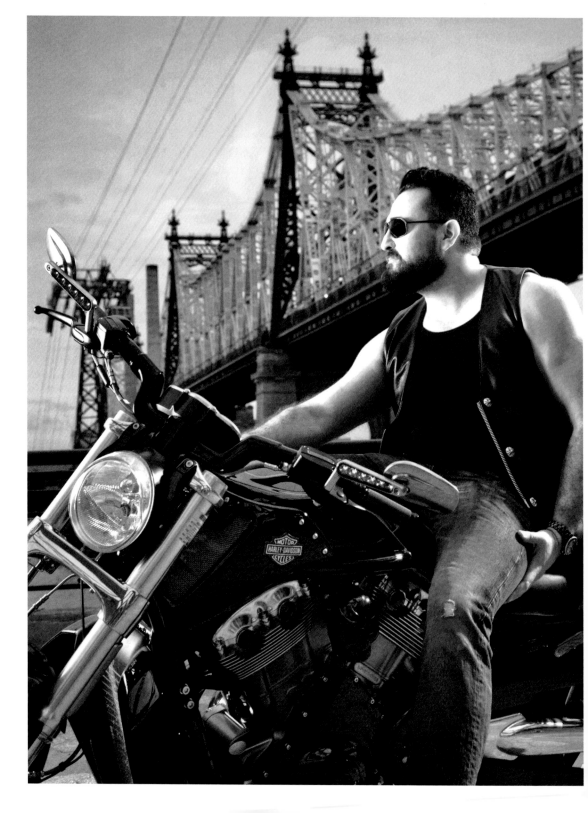

ACKNOWLEDGMENTS

The writing and development of **MANMADE** has been the culmination of a long-time dream and the start of a new journey. This process has allowed me to share both what I have learned through many years of work and what so many men have taught me along the way. It has also given me the gift of editing down, focusing, and refining what I believe really matters. We are in an exciting time as men, and the rules that once confined us are no longer in our way.

While this book has been an absolute labor of love, it is not one I could have accomplished alone. Like any leader, I have had the incredible good fortune of being surrounded by exceptional teams at every turn. That includes my entire team at Kiehl's Since 1851, past and present, that continuously inspires me. I'd like to thank Rob Imig, Lauren Rodolitz, Zoey Larsen, Maria Gustafson, Christina Gabriel, and Candida Junor for helping me fine-tune my ideas for **MANMADE**. My incredible mentors and L'Oréal family have been tremendously supportive, most specifically Jean-Paul Agon, Nicolas Hieronimus, Laurent Attal, and Marc Menesguen. I want to extend special gratitude to Frederic Roze and Carol Hamilton for always believing in me.

My codreamers at Davis Brand Capital have been counselors and creators who served me particularly well: Teri Schindler, Eleanor Safe, Manon Herzog, Bryan Oekel, Bruce Burton, Alison Doerfler, Mason Clark, Blair Smith, and especially Patrick Davis, to whom I am eternally grateful for partnering with me on the incredible journey of **MANMADE**. And, of course, the outstanding team at Penguin Random House, most notably the inimitable Pam Krauss and her exceptional team, including Nina Caldas, Ian Dingman, Robert Siek, and Derek Gullino. I am so very honored to be part of the first list from Pam Krauss Books.

My thanks would be incomplete without particular recognition of the men who helped me make this book a record of real life: Anthony Mackie, Teddy Sears, Paul Cox, Grant Reynolds, James Cayzer (Jaytech), and Jake Barton. I'm grateful for their generosity in sharing their time and experience with me and all those who read **MANMADE**.

Finally, to my family, personal friends, and trusted advisers: I could not have done this—or anything else—without your wisdom, patience, trust, belief, or love. I am humbled by all you have given me along the way.

INDEX

ABOUT THE AUTHOR

CHRIS SALGARDO is a long-time beauty and skincare executive who has worked for Chanel, Inc., Estée Lauder Companies, and L'Oréal USA. Salgardo has a never-ending curiosity about grooming, skincare, and how to put your best face forward. He is a powerful example of business success achieved through genuine passion. A board member of RxArt and a donor to amfAR for more than two decades, Salgardo is an avid philanthropist. He is currently president of the iconic Kiehl's Since 1851 brand in the United States.